MARK ANTHONY'S
ONCE-A-WEEK
WORKOUT

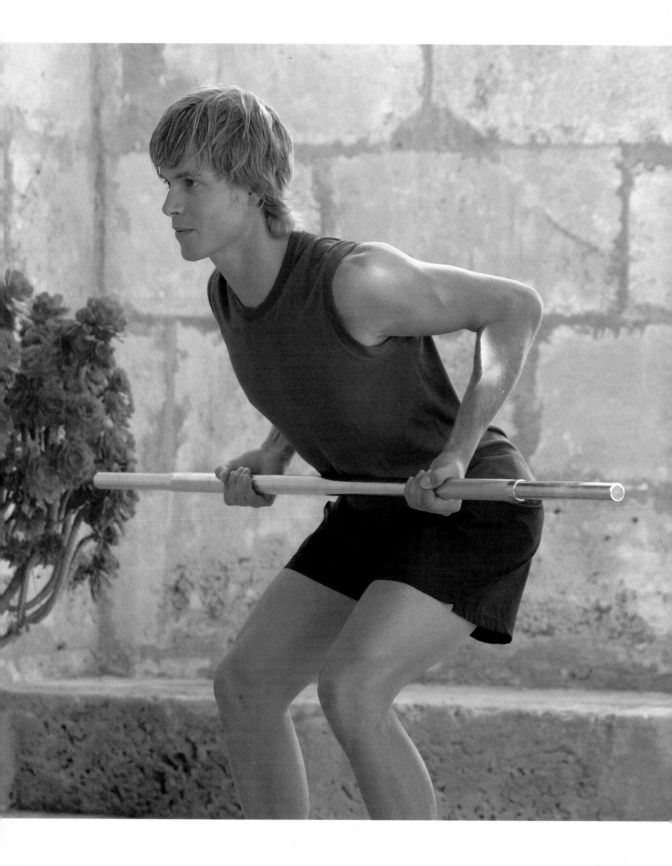

MARK ANTHONY'S
ONCE-A-WEEK WORKOUT

Transform your body in 12 weeks

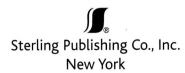

Sterling Publishing Co., Inc.
New York

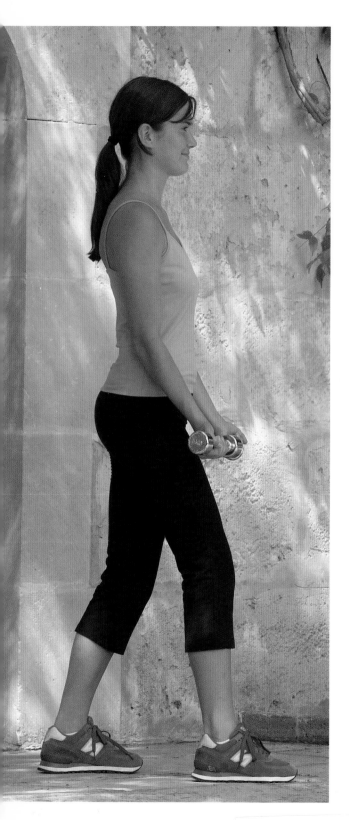

For my Gillian, my Luke, and
my Sophie, I love you guys.

Library of Congress Cataloging-in-Publication Data Available

10 9 8 7 6 5 4 3 2 1

Published in 2006 by Sterling Publishing Co., Inc.
387 Park Avenue South, New York, NY 10016

First published in 2006 by Collins & Brown,
An imprint of Chrysalis Books Group plc
The Chrysalis Building, Bramley Road, London W10 6SP
Text © 2006 by Mark Anthony
Photographs © 2006 by Collins & Brown

Distributed in Canada by Sterling Publishing
C/o Canadian Manda Group, 165 Dufferin Street
Toronto, Ontario, Canada M6K 3H6

Printed in China

Sterling ISBN-13: 978-1-4027-3748-0
        ISBN-10: 1-4027-3748-3

For information about custom editions, special sales,
premium and corporate purchases, please contact
Sterling Special Sales Department at 800-805-5489 or
specialsales@sterlingpub.com.

Contents

Introduction

The world of fitness is full of contradictions. We are presented with endless possibilities and options. Often it is only instinct that leads us to our chosen path. But how do we sift through media confusion, the many exercise theories offered, and fad diets? Let me simplify it for you.

Through my experience and research, I can tell you that scientific evidence shows that it is intensity, rather than frequency or volume, which is the major factor in achieving fitness.

My father was a sprinter, my grandfather a supreme gymnast, my uncle Duncan a champion boxer, and my uncle Aiden Mr. Great Britain and an Olympic weightlifting Gold medalist. As you can see, fitness runs through my veins.

I have been fortunate enough to have personally trained more than a thousand individuals, starting at large health and fitness organizations, and now at my studio in London. During this time, my knowledge and experience in personal training have come together to produce *Once-a-Week Workout*. The countless hours of working with people on a one-to-one basis, is still a tremendous thrill for me. Actually watching someone progress way past their own expectations is the ultimate in job satisfaction.

Due to the many stress factors, as well as time and economic restraints in our society today, most people find it impossible to commit to a 3-day-a-week exercise program. My research and study cases show that the clients who worked hard and trained for 3 days a week found it impossible to sustain their fitness program. Time constraints and everyday pressures, combined with overexercise can lead to exhaustion; therefore the majority of people give up.

My once-a-week workout will leave you feeling completely energized and full of enthusiasm as a result of focusing all your energy into one, intense workout a week. I have created the formula for a totally balanced lifestyle, which I would like to share with you.

Nothing burns body fat in the same way as resistance training, and that is why it is possible for the human body to change so dramatically over such a short period of time, using my workout, an active lifestyle, and a healthy diet. My "Total Body Development System" combines every segment of fitness, strength, stamina, speed, flexibility, and appetite, creating a formula for success that I call "The Fitness Circle."

So if you dislike the body you're in, want to rapidly reduce fat and cellulite, want to drop 2 dress sizes and lose up to 24lb (11kg) in 3 months, changing your life forever; prepare to embark on a series of workouts that will enhance the performance of your body, over a 12-week period, with startling results.

In 4 weeks I'll change the way you feel about exercising. In 8 weeks I'll change your body. In 12 weeks I'll change your life. Is it possible? You bet!

Mark Anthony
www.thefitnesscircle.co.uk

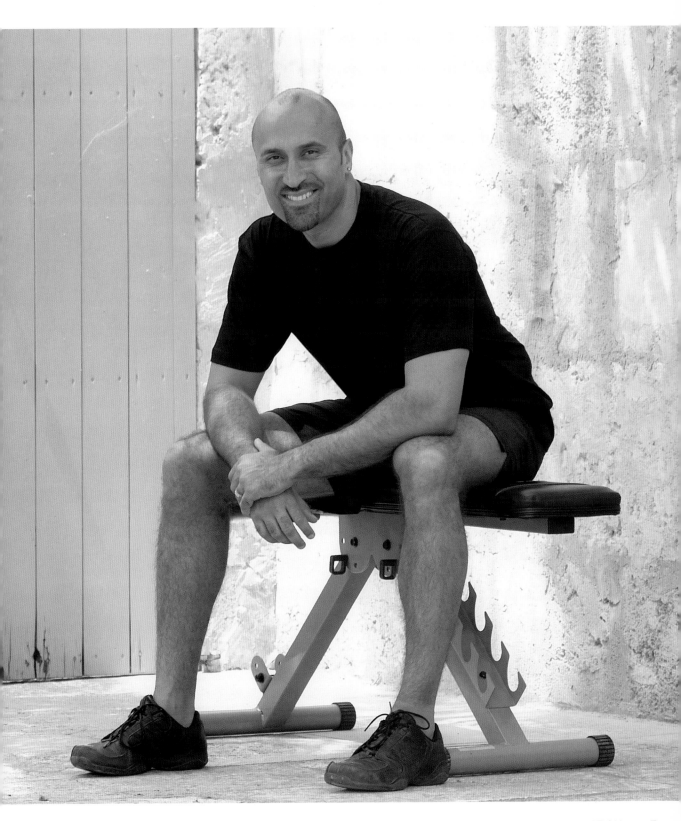

The Fitness Circle

STRENGTH   FLEXIBILITY

STAMINA   NUTRITION

SPEED

Medical Questionnaire

	Do you suffer from back pain?
	Are you suffering from a long-term illness?
	Do you have high blood pressure?
	Have you had surgery over the past 2 years?
	Do you suffer from high cholesterol?
	Are you pregnant?
	Do you drink an excessive amount of alcohol?
	Do you smoke?
	Do you have tension or soreness in a specific area?
	Do you suffer from chest pains?
	Have you sustained an injury over the past 3 months?
	Do you suffer from any other joint problem?
	Has any member of your family had any form of heart complaint?
	If you have ticked any of the above, please consult your doctor before starting the program .

CASE STUDY 1: Susan Vriesman (42 yrs)

I first started Mark Anthony's fitness program about 8 months after the birth of my second child. I had thought about going to a gym when my first child was born 5 years ago, but that was as far as it got. When I read about Mark's 12-week program it was enough to make me pick up the phone and call him. Mark was very approachable and asked me about my last workout—about 20 years ago—then a few other questions and an appointment was made.

The dreaded day came when I was weighed, asked about my eating habits (OK-ish!), my drinking habits (too much beer), and my exercise regime (nothing—apart from looking after two young children!) Then came the scary part: starting the exercise regime! I managed to crawl on the treadmill, try a few very weak lunges (with no weights apart from my excess body weight), and lift a few weights to try to strengthen my upper body.

Miraculously after only 4 weeks I already felt better. I had lost several pounds and inches. Encouraged by this my diet improved, I watched my fat intake and ate more fruit and salads, and even began to enjoy drinking 3 ½ pints (2 liters) of water a day.

At the end of 12 weeks my weight loss was an amazing 28lb (12.6kg), and my dress size down from a generous size 10 to a small size 6. Apart from looking better, my energy levels have increased considerably.

A year on and I still train with Mark once a week and have never felt so good. I can now run on the treadmill and lunge with 17.5lb (8kg) in each hand, which was almost my total weight loss.

I have never had so many compliments on my appearance; my husband loves the new me, even though he had to buy me a complete new wardrobe.

I cannot believe what a difference Mark's fitness program has made to me. I look forward to my weekly workouts, and leave it feeling exhilarated.

This exercise program, following a healthier lifestyle, and Mark's encouragement and enthusiasm have made a huge impact on both me and my family.

MARK'S COMMENTS

Susan's commitment to her exercise is the reason why she looks amazing. For anyone to lose 28lb over 12 weeks is a remarkable achievement. To change somebody's habits is extremely difficult, and implementing a structured, new lifestyle can be daunting. But once you've cracked it, your whole outlook on yourself totally changes. Your movement becomes better. You're able to keep up with the kids and you become stronger mentally and physically. Focus all your energy in one space during one hour of exercise, and make the change in yourself, as Susan has forever.

"We are always learning. With exercise, knowledge itself is not enough. You must apply what you believe in. Only through this can you achieve success."

Just once a week...

Obesity is a worldwide epidemic that is growing rapidly. Twenty percent of the world's population is clinically obese, and fifty percent is seriously overweight.

Weight loss and fitness enhancement is what most of us want to achieve from an exercise program. The *Once-a-Week Workout* allows this to happen at a steady rate. The key to keeping the weight off permanently is to lose 2.2lb (1kg) of fat per week. Muscle weighs more than fat, so although this may seem a relatively small amount to lose on a weekly basis, 2.2lb (1kg) per week is equal to 30lb (13.6kg), of fat over a 12-week period. You try putting that back on—no chance!

Aerobic activity burns, on average, 200 to 550 calories per hour. In comparison, high-intensity resistance training burns $3^{1}/_{2}$ times that amount. For optimal weight loss, the scale of activity must outweigh the amount of calories consumed above your body's basic metabolic rate. Your weight in kg x 20 = equals the amount of calories needed at rest.

Psychologically, it is hard to convince yourself that exercising with resistance only once a week can actually make a difference to your body, health, and overall fitness. But you'd be surprised. As a personal trainer, l have studied the effects of overtraining or exercising three to four times a week. It has a detrimental effect on the body, causing fatigue, depression, irritability, increased injuries, chronic muscle soreness, excessive weight loss, frequent minor infections, and appetite loss. These factors occur because most of us apply high-intensity training to nearly all of our workouts. The body can't cope with this! A regime like this is also extremely difficult to commit to long-term. Your once-a-week workout, however, can be effortlessly implemented into your weekly schedule. Weight training should be done infrequently so that your muscles can regenerate and heal, allowing for increased lean muscle and increased metabolism.

Exercise helps your body produce endorphins, providing you with the feel-good factor and loads of energy. It increases self-confidence and promotes libido. Question yourself: How many times am I currently going to the gym, and have l seen any results over the past 12 months?

What we are going to achieve is maximum results over a short period of time, increased stamina, strength, tone and lean muscle, and decreased blood pressure, resting heart rate, and body fat.

The science

The human body is like a tree. For it to form properly, both the base and core of the tree have to be strong. Once that is achieved, everything else blossoms. l used this principle when creating the workouts.

The key is to train the largest muscles—the legs—first. They demand the greatest amount of oxygen because they are the largest muscle group. Then move on to the back, the pectorals, shoulders, triceps, biceps, and finally the abdomen. Always concentrate on drawing in the abdominal muscles and focus on good posture.

By working the entire body during one workout, we maximize calorie burning. The idea is to try to work at a pace that allows you to train the body in a certain way, reducing rest periods

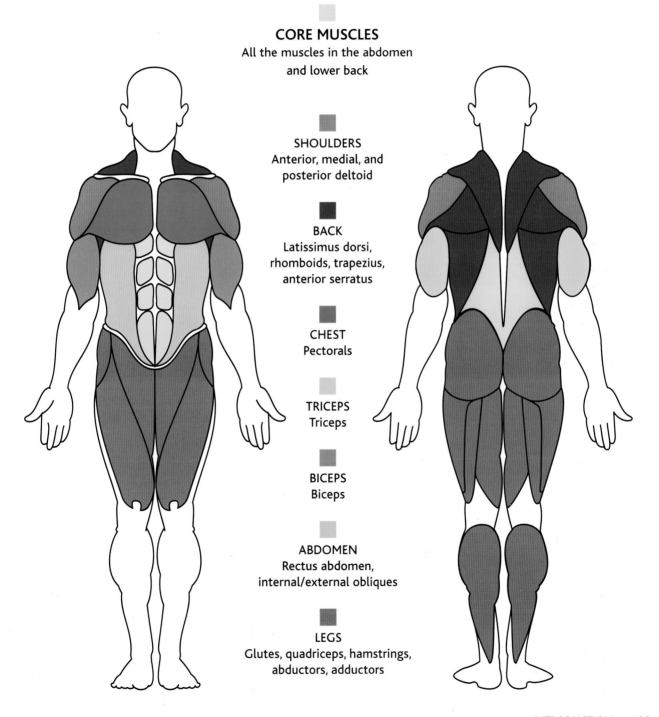

CORE MUSCLES
All the muscles in the abdomen
and lower back

SHOULDERS
Anterior, medial, and
posterior deltoid

BACK
Latissimus dorsi,
rhomboids, trapezius,
anterior serratus

CHEST
Pectorals

TRICEPS
Triceps

BICEPS
Biceps

ABDOMEN
Rectus abdomen,
internal/external obliques

LEGS
Glutes, quadriceps, hamstrings,
abductors, adductors

in between sets and exercises. This keeps the heart rate elevated, and the entire workout is set at high intensity, which enhances fat burning!

I have always found rhythmical repetitions to be the safest and fastest way of exercise to build strength, and the best form to isolate individual muscle fibers in the body. The repetitions permit maximum muscle contractions throughout the full range of joint movement. So it's irrelevant how much weight you lift, the speed of the repetition should always remain the same: two seconds up, two seconds down! The art of performing a set of one exercise is not to go too fast, but to allow the muscles to do the work: a set of 8 to 12 repetitions are commonly used to increase lean muscle. The upper body responds well with this repetition range, but the lower body responds far better with slightly higher repetitions. The body doesn't seem to be satisfied with just one set, so the first set is always used as a secondary warm up, which also prevents injury. It's the second set of the exercise that is the challenge, and the goal: to complete the desired number of repetitions, all using good technique during the set of an exercise. So, come on, pump it out!

The mind is a powerful tool. Try to establish a link between the mind and muscle connection, and feel each repetition of the working set.

Visualization is a strong principle to use both during and after exercise, and it's amazing how the human body adapts to physical stress so quickly. So always try and progress and overload the workout on a weekly basis. Power comes from breathing within, so remember to breathe constantly during the exercises. Whether it's a pull, push, or press, try to breathe out on the exertion.

Rest and recuperation are vital after intense exercise. However, it is now the norm to rest for 48 hours and perform the same program again. With this kind of regime, however, it is neither possible or necessary.

When you perform constructive exercise with resistance, your muscle fibers need to heal and regenerate so that they become stronger. After high-intensity resistance work, seven days rest is required for your muscle fibers to fully heal, form, and become stronger, allowing you optimal performance during your weekly workouts. The stronger you are, the leaner you will become. By allowing your body ample rest from intense work, we can incorporate cardiovascular activity, exercising at a much lower rate of intensity, strengthening your heart and lungs, and also enhancing the prospect of fat burning! Our bodies like this form of exercise mainly because it's so much easier to perform.

Walking, running, and cycling, for instance, are all forms of cardio lifestyles that we can easily fit in to our busy schedules. These activities can be done on a daily basis. If you incorporate just two or three cardio lifestyles around the once-a-week workout, you will successfully achieve complete fitness.

CASE STUDY 2: Anna Sljivic (35 yrs)

I started working out with Mark in January 2005. I had been working out regularly since my mid-twenties but had begun to lose my motivation over the past year and was working increasingly longer hours, the combination of which resulted in fewer and fewer workouts. I realized I would be turning 35 shortly and knew that it would be increasingly easier (under inertia) to continue the downhill trend while work-related stress was on the increase. I needed a boost and sought out Mark.

I've always enjoyed exercising but, while I was fairly fit, I knew I had a few pockets of body fat that I was quite adept at concealing. I remember thinking at the time that Mark's claim of "changing my life" after 12 weeks was rather ambitious but I figured I had nothing to lose. In fact, by week three, I felt that he had already changed my life. Of course, after only two workouts, the visible physical changes were still only beginning to emerge, but I noticed an unprecedented psychological change. I had renewed vigor and enthusiasm and my mood was completely transformed. This has only increased. I have to attribute this change to the intensity of each workout and Mark's relentlessness as a trainer. It is incredible how effective a 60-minute workout can be, particularly since I, like many, had typically done 2–3 workouts per week yet was always "saving myself" for fear of overdoing it. Mark is totally focused on maximizing each second of time and his pre-fatiguing technique pushes me to my limits but still leaves me some ability to crawl out of his studio at the end of it. It feels each time like I am transcending my own abilities, and this is a tremendously empowering feeling.

On the physical side, the results have been no less dramatic. My body fat went down from 27 percent to 24 percent in the first five weeks; by the end of six months it was at 18 percent. From week to week, I have noticed the appearance of new muscles. Mark is nothing short of a magician. He not only transforms bodies but he and his methodology have such a huge impact on one's psyche that working out with him truly is a life-changing experience.

MARK'S COMMENTS

When I first met Anna she found resistance work testing. The introduction to squats and upper body movements with minimum rest periods enabled her entire body to wake up. Now she looks fantastic! Together we have worked so hard on developing her legs and glutes, the end result being a beautifully balanced body. Anna's abs are so well developed that she constantly exercises with a confident smile, which shows just how pleased she is with herself. Having fun with exercise is a must, especially when you can see results as Anna has!

"I exercise each week for purpose, pleasure, and fulfillment. Exercise for me is freedom of mind. It is my time of selfishness."

1. Graph showing an individual's increased strength on a bench press over 12 weeks

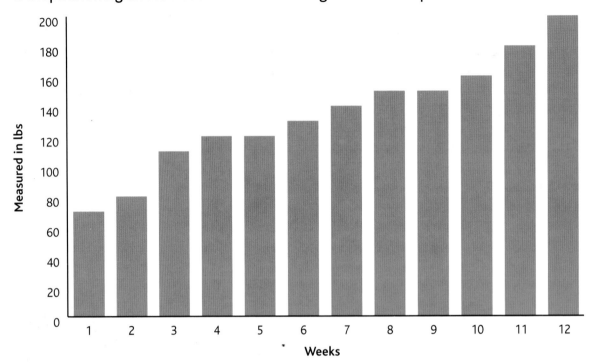

2. Graph showing the reduction of body fat in an individual over a period of 12 weeks

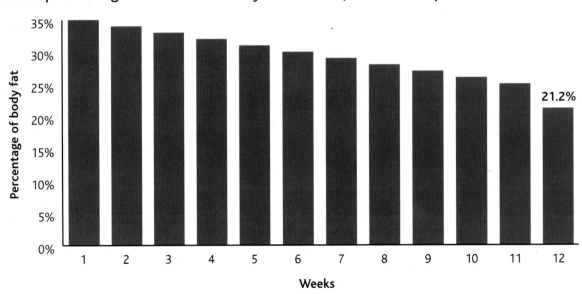

1. Graph showing increased strength

This graph shows an individual's performance on a bench press. By not implementing further resistance work during the same week, this particular person became stronger and stronger on a weekly basis. The body builds through memory and experience and being competitive with oneself is a good thing. It is true to say that you only get out what you put in, staying true to the old saying, "no pain no gain." So, challenge your body and allow it to respond.

2. Graph showing reduced body fat

This shows a 50-year-old female's body fat levels slowly decreasing over the 12-week period. She achieved excellent results and a totally balanced lifestyle. Balance is happiness. It is you in control of your body and overall well-being. Don't forget, your health is your wealth.

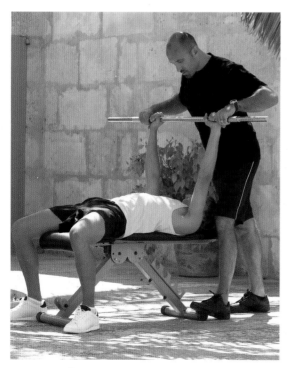

Two-arm chest press with barbell

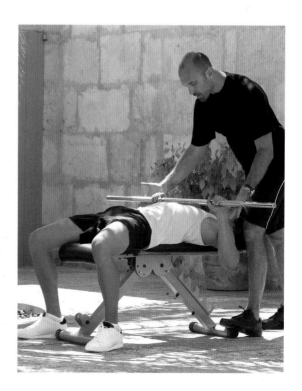

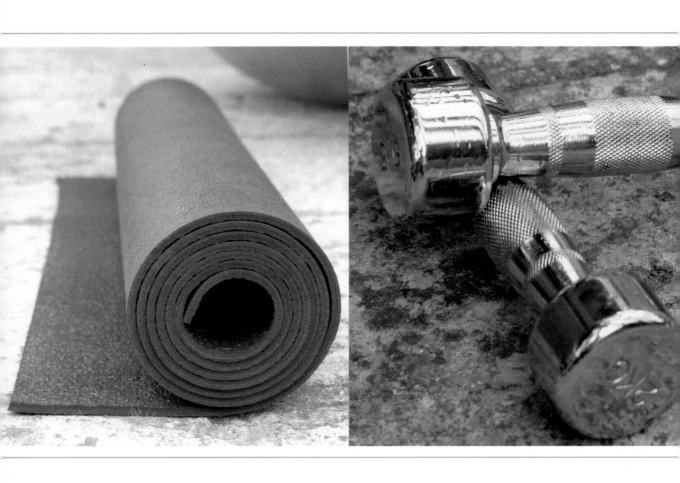

Equipment 1

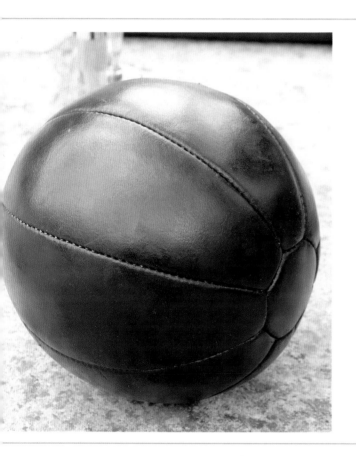

Although it is possible that you could use water bottles instead of dumbbells, a chair in place of a stability ball, and a flat surface with a head support instead of a multiangle bench, for the best results it really is worth investing in the right equipment. Interchangeable dumbbells are superb for speed between sets, and a nonslip stability ball works best with all exercises. A pedometer and heart-rate monitor are also worth considering for all other activities.

Let's make a start

Your once-a-week workout starts here! Select a day in the week that you can try to keep as your "training day," adding optional cardio activities around it. Don't forget that this is your hour. You'll find that having a tremendous workout will make you feel full of energy, especially after the best part—the shower! What a feeling!

Before starting the workout, select a comfortable weight that you feel you can use while performing all the exercises. You need to experience what it feels like to train at high intensity with the exact rest periods in between.

The beginning stage requires 40 seconds rest between exercises. As you progress throughout your 12-week cycle, the rest periods decrease to 30 seconds in weeks 5 to 8 and down to just 20 seconds for weeks 9 to 12. You will notice that there are some exercises in the workout called *Supersets*. These require the individual to complete an exercise and immediately follow the first exercise with another exercise that works the same muscle group.

There are 12 exercises at the beginner's stage, weeks 1 to 4. There are 14 exercises for the intermediate level at weeks 5 to 8, and 16 exercises for the advanced level at weeks 9 to 12. The beginner workout is an initial trial test for you. Use the same resistance to perform both sets of an exercise to start with. Only increase the resistance once you've achieved 12 repetitions on the second set.

From this, you should distinguish which exercises are hard, and which are easy, so that you can set the resistance to suit. Make sure you are well hydrated before your workout, and if you feel unwell during exercise, please stop.

Equipment

1. Stability ball
This maximizes core stabilization, is great for posture correction, abdominal work, and helps correct your form and technique for each exercise.

2. Medicine ball
This is a great bit of kit! Alternatively use a soccer ball. It is excellent for exercises that involve the entire body, and also isolation exercises that target specific muscles, such as the abdomen.

3. Dumbbells.
I love training with dumbbells. These tools are responsible for shaping and conditioning the entire body through different angles of exercise.

4. Barbell
A lot of people shy away from using a barbell, but for exercises that produce results, such as the reverse barbell row, this tool works really well.

5. Matting
This is imperative for safety. It provides a platform that prevents you from slipping during exercises such as lunges. It is also essential for performing abdominal and stretching exercises.

6. Multiangle weight-training bench
This can be used flat, at a low-level incline, and high-level incline. Use it for numerous exercises working the entire body. This is an essential piece of kit that provides valuable body support.

If you cannot find any of the equipment above, you can use 16-oz water bottles instead of dumbbells, a chair instead of a stability ball, and a flat surface with a head support instead of a bench. Ideally, for great results, invest in the right equipment.

The art of motivation is vital to exercise. Achieving what you want, not just with fitness and body change, but in all other aspects of your life, requires motivation and discipline. After the first workout, remember what you did and how you felt afterward. After workout 12, think about what you have achieved!

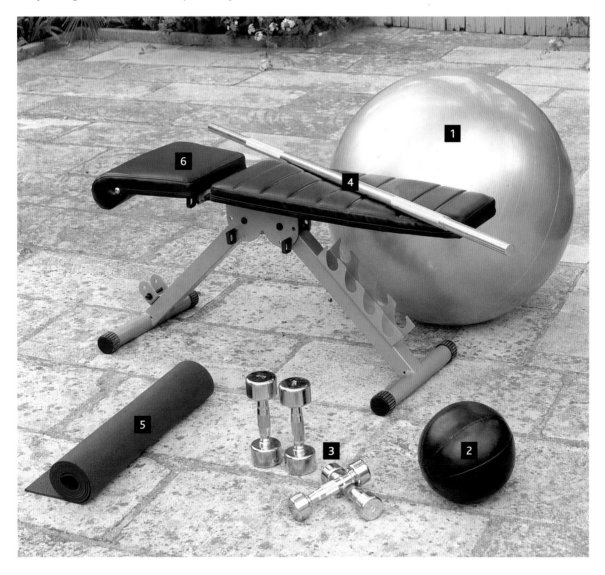

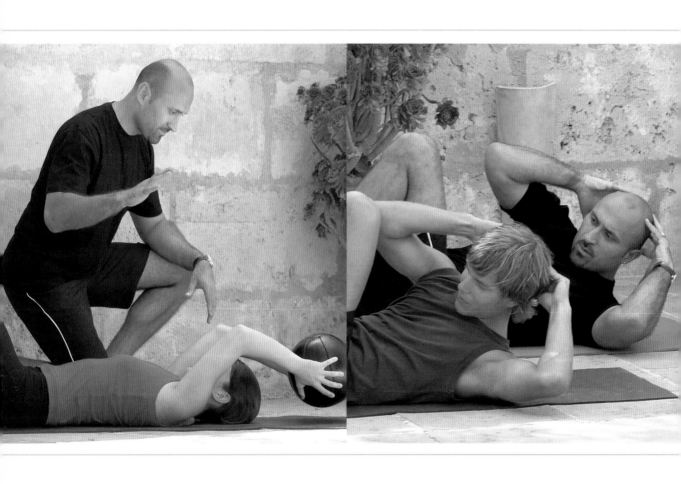

The Once-a-Week Workouts 2

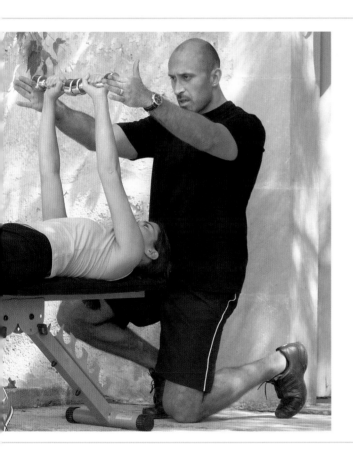

Think about how you want your body to look and set personal goals. Now put all your energy into your weekly workouts, and whenever possible increase resistance. You need to make this change and I know you want to. Tone up, lose fat, and sculpt your body. Visualize that thought every time you approach your weekly workouts! This is your chance to embrace the fitness circle lifestyle. Remember, don't touch any weights afterward for another seven days. Enjoy!

The warm-up

Performing light activity raises the body's temperature and warms your muscles for strength training. Your joints become mobilized, and because you've successfully warmed up, your body's ready for constructive exercise. Always warm up at a rate that suits you. A warm-up can be made up of running on the spot, throwing a ball with a partner, a six-minute walk, or as I prefer, using a medicine ball. Activate your core muscles by focusing and pulling your navel into your spine.

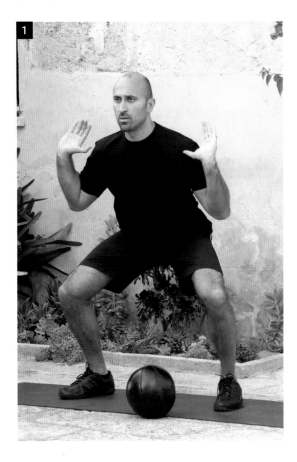

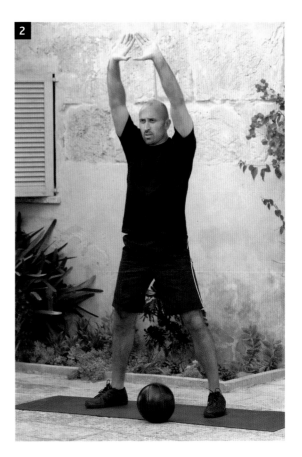

1 With your stance at shoulder width, toes pointing outward, activate your core muscles. Place your hands on either side of your collarbone, palms facing away from you. Squat down so you are parallel to the floor, keeping your back straight.

2 Now press upward, allowing your hands to reach above you, and stand tall. Instantly move into the start position and repeat this movement 20 times.

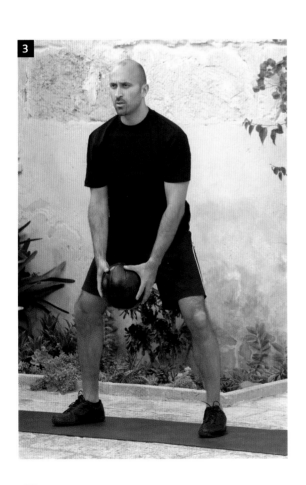

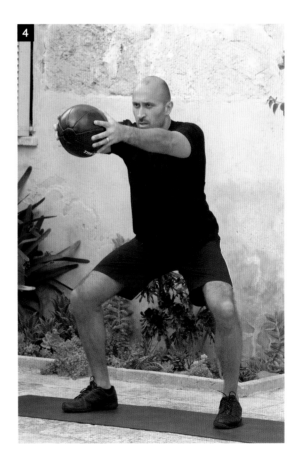

3 Now grasp a medicine ball. Keeping your elbows soft, activate your core muscles. Bend at the knees, keeping your neck relaxed.

4 Now drop down into a squat position keeping your back straight and raise the ball with both arms in front of you. Return to the start position and repeat the movement 20 times. Now repeat the entire warm-up sequence twice.

1 Beginner workout for women

Allow 40 seconds rest between each exercise and try to move quickly between sets. Make sure to keep the speed of the repetitions 2 seconds up, 2 seconds down!

Squat with stability ball   2 Sets 12 Reps

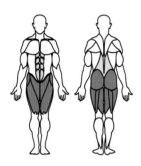

The muscles being worked here are the quads, hamstrings, and glutes. Focus on the muscles you are working. Make sure you squeeze those glutes.

1 Place the stability ball behind you, against a wall. Walk your feet away so that you are leaning into the ball with your stance at shoulder width, arms outstretched in front of you. Activate your core muscles.

2 Perform a squat and bend at the knees so that your hips are parallel to the ground. Press upward back to the starting position and repeat.

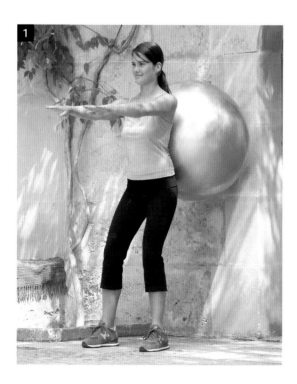

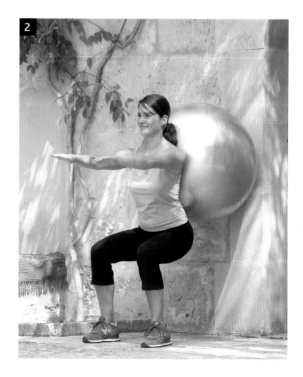

Two-point alternate lunges 2 Sets 15 Reps

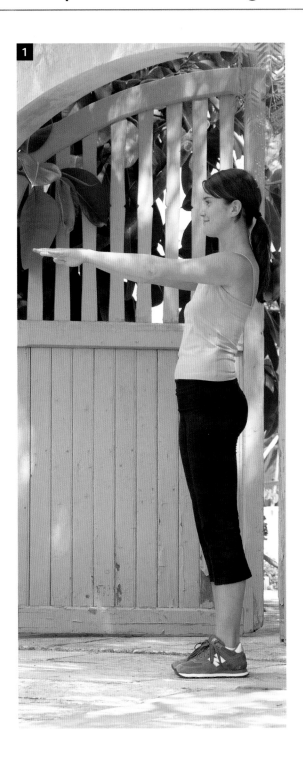

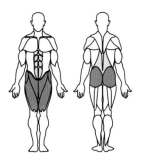

This is such a good exercise for the fronts of your thighs! Try to get a rhythm going and remember, good form is essential for good development and condition.

1 Start in an upright position, arms straight out in front of you. Activate your core muscles.

2 Step forward with one leg bending at the hips, knee, and ankle. Push upward and change legs, performing the same movement.

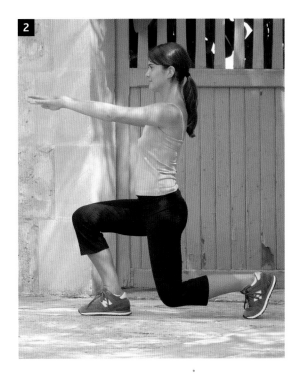

Squat and press with dumbbells 2 Sets 15 Reps

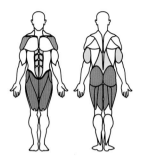

The muscles being worked here are the quads, hamstrings, glutes, deltoids, and triceps. Don't rush this exercise. Try to keep to the 2 seconds up, 2 seconds down rule.

1 From a standing position with soft knees, grasp a set of dumbbells and bring your hands up on either side of your collarbone, with the palms of your hands facing away from you. Activate your core muscles.

2 With your stance at shoulder width, squat down bending at the knees.

3 Press upward with the glutes, and in doing so, also press the dumbbells above your head. Lower the dumbbells under control, and swiftly repeat the sequence. Don't quit on me!

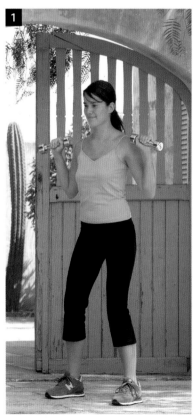

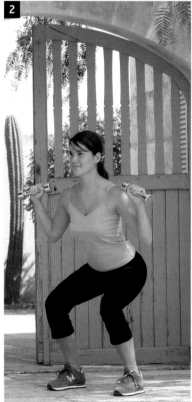

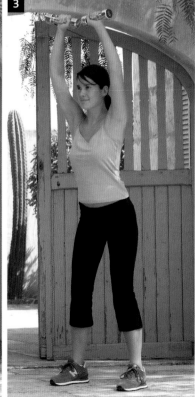

Row with medicine ball   2 Sets 12 Reps

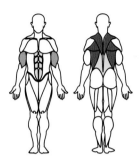

The muscles being worked are the latissimus dorsi, rhomboids, trapezius, and biceps. Maintain a straight back throughout the movement, and focus on the working muscles in the back. Keep that ball pumping!

1 From a standing position, stance at hip width, grasp a medicine ball or soccer ball. Activate your core muscles. Lean forward, keeping your back straight, and your arms at length.

2 Under control, pull the ball in toward you, driving the elbows back and squeezing your shoulder blades together. Lower the resistance under control, and repeat the sequence. Each repetition counts!

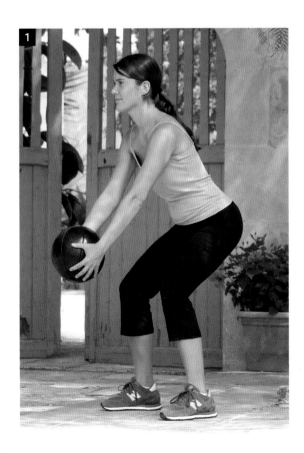

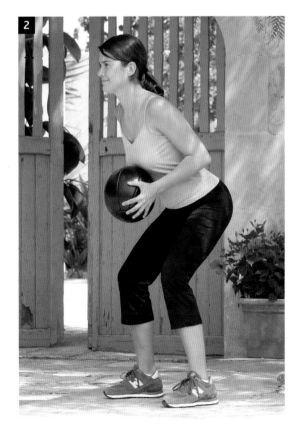

Seated bench row 2 Sets 12 Reps

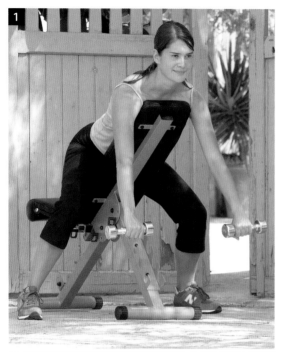

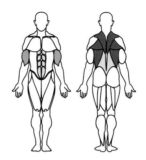

The muscles being worked are the latissimus dorsi, rhomboids, trapezius, and biceps. This is such a good exercise for your back. Having the bench set at 45 degrees provides you with the right angle to perform the exercise without cheating.

1 On an incline bench, grasp hold of a set of dumbbells, with the palms of your hands facing toward you and your arms out at full length. Sit on the bench so that your chest is against the incline pad. Activate your core muscles.

2 Pull the dumbbells in toward you, so that they are either side of your chest. Under control, lower to the start position and repeat. Focus on your breathing!

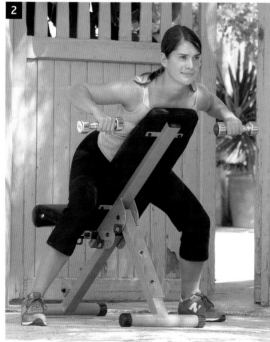

Two-arm flat chest press with dumbbells 2 Sets 12 Reps

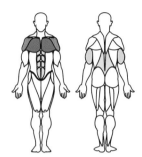

The muscles being worked are the pectorals, deltoids, and triceps. Feel your chest muscles contract and link the mind and muscle together.

1 Grasping a set of dumbbells, lie on a flat bench. Activate your core muscles. Press the dumbbells up with the elbows to the sides, until the arms are extended.

2 Under control, lower the weights to the sides of the chest. Push the dumbbells away from your chest until the arms are straight but not locked. Repeat the sequence.

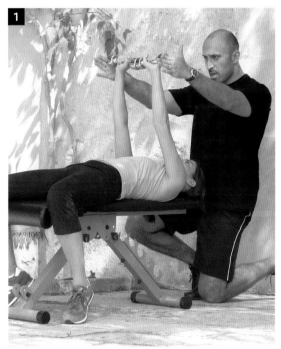

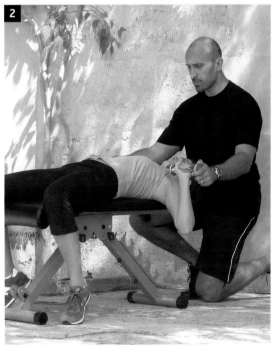

Shoulder press on a stability ball with dumbbells   2 Sets 12 Reps

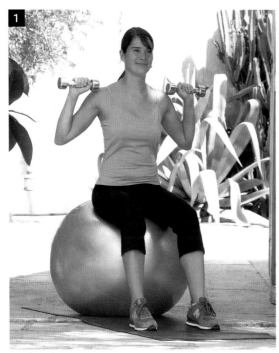

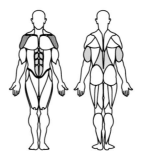

The muscles being worked are the deltoids and the triceps. Press using your shoulders and the backs of your arms. Isolate these muscles and stay focused!

1 Sitting on a stability ball, maintain a stable posture keeping your back straight. Grasp a set of dumbbells and activate your core muscles.

2 With the dumbbells on either side of your collarbone, palms facing away from you, press upward. Make sure to keep the arms straight, but not locked. Under control, lower the dumbbells back to the start position and repeat the movement.

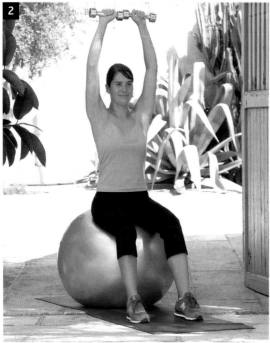

Two-arm triceps extension with dumbbells 2 Sets 12 Reps

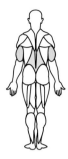

The muscles being worked on are the triceps. Try to keep the shoulders totally still during this exercise, and make those muscles work!

1 Lying on a flat bench, grasp a set of dumbbells. Activate your core muscles. Press both dumbbells in front of you with the palms of your hands facing each other.

2 Bend only from the elbows, allowing the dumbbells to go past your head and in line with your ears. Push upward, and contract your triceps muscles.

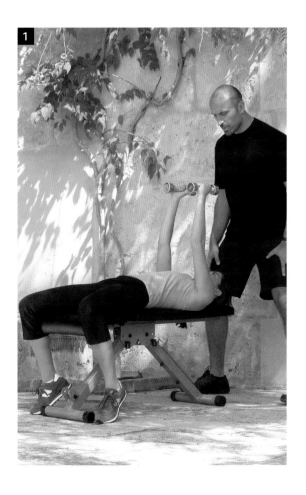

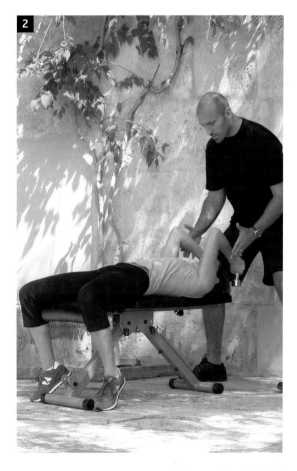

Two-arm standing biceps curl with barbell 2 Sets 15 Reps

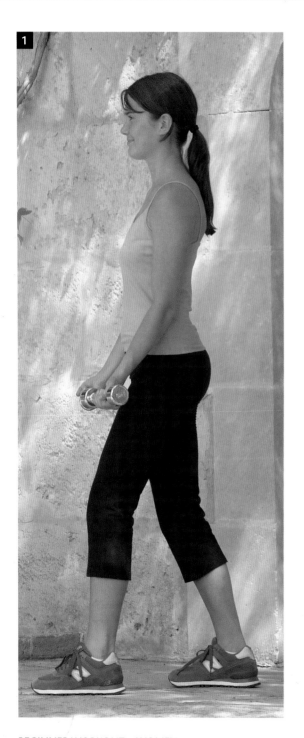

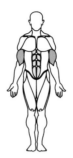

The muscles being worked on here are the biceps. Squeeze the them at the top. Always keep the elbows soft through the full range of joint movement.

1 From a standing position, left leg forward, right leg back, grasp a barbell with your palms facing away from you.

2 Keeping the elbows locked into the sides, bend the elbow joints and perform a curl. Lower the weight under control and repeat the movement.

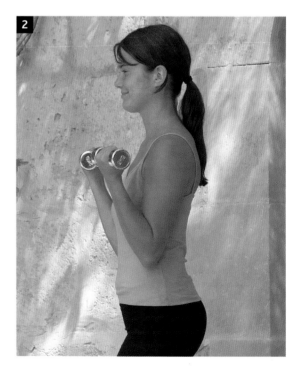

Reaches 2 Sets 20 Reps

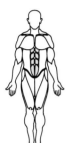

The muscles being worked are the rectus abdomen. Maintain the speed of your repetitions, 2 seconds up, 2 seconds down. Feel the abs burn!

1 Lying flat on an exercise mat, bend at the knees and lift your heels. Activate your core muscles. Lengthen both arms in front of you, so that they are in line with your shoulders.

2 Raise your head and shoulder blades off the floor, allowing the abdomen to contract. Lower under control and repeat. Keep the movement smooth and rhythmical.

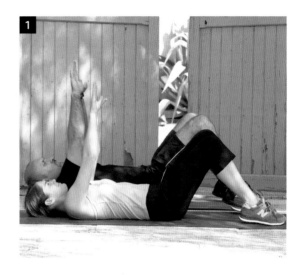

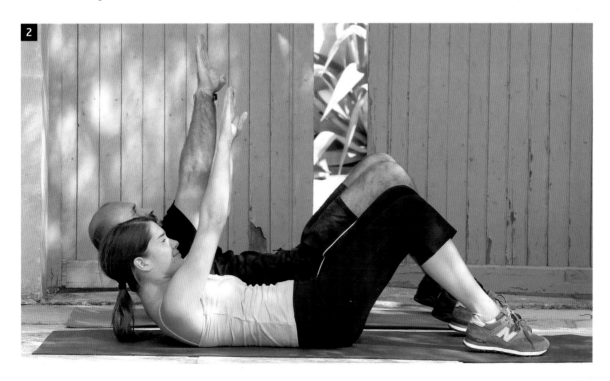

Crocodile crunch   2 Sets 20 Reps

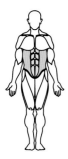

In this exercise the muscle being worked is the rectus abdomen. Go for it! Stop and I'll make you do it all over again!

1 Lying on a mat, lift both legs toward you with hips and knees in line. Activate your core muscles.

2 With your head and neck off the floor, raise the upper torso, and at the same time bring your legs toward you. Now reach. Lower under control and repeat the movement. Come on!

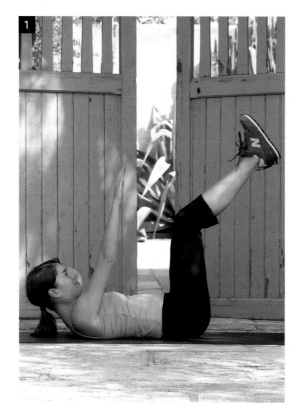

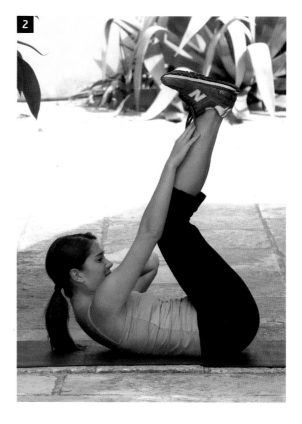

The plank 2 Sets 20 Second hold

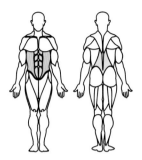

The entire core area is being worked here. Try to breathe normally when doing this challenging exercise and focus on tightening your core muscles.

1 Activate your core muscles, drawing your navel to your spine. Resting on your forearms and toes, hold your body up. Keep your elbows under your shoulder blades with your forearms facing forward.

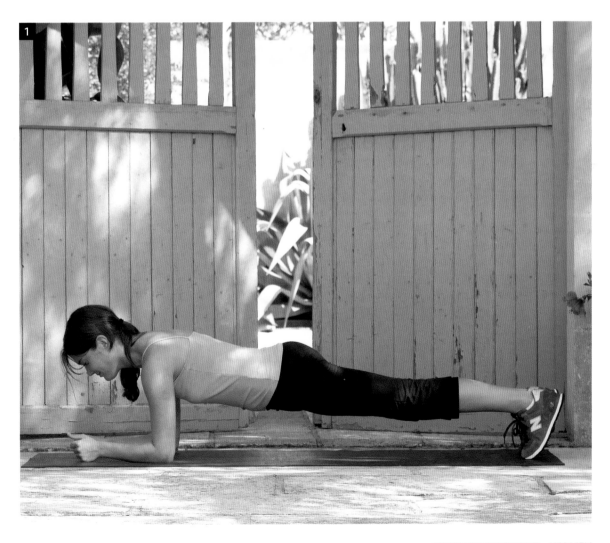

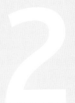

Beginner workout for men

Allow 40 seconds rest between each exercise and try to move quickly between sets. Make sure to keep the speed of the repetitions 2 seconds up, 2 seconds down!

Squat with stability ball and dumbbells 2 Sets 15 Reps

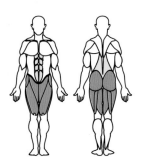

The muscles being worked here are the quads, hamstrings, and glutes. Press through the glutes and always keep the movement under control.

1 Place the stability ball behind you, against a wall. Grasp the dumbbells either side of you, with palms facing each other. Activate your core muscles, navel to spine. Walk your feet away so that you are leaning into the ball, stance at shoulder width.

2 Perform a squat, and bend at the knees so that your hips are parallel to the ground. Press upward, back to the starting position.

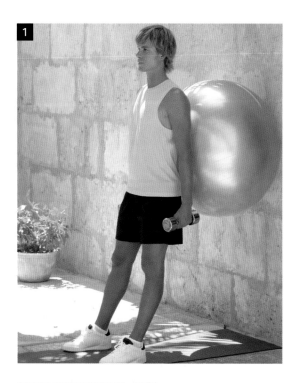

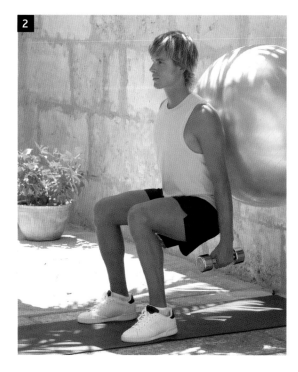

Dead-lift with dumbbells 2 Sets 15 Reps

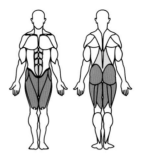

The muscles being worked are the glutes and quadriceps. Remember to keep your elbows and knees soft while performing any resistance-based movement.

1 From a standing position, stance at hip width, grasp a set of dumbbells with your palms facing you, and activate your core muscles.

2 Bend from the hips and knees keeping your back straight and your arms at length. Push through the glutes and return to the start position.

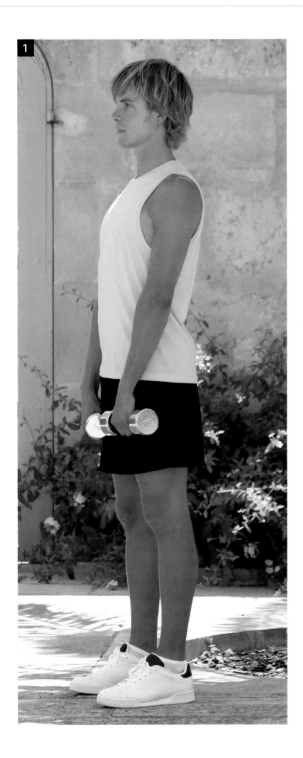

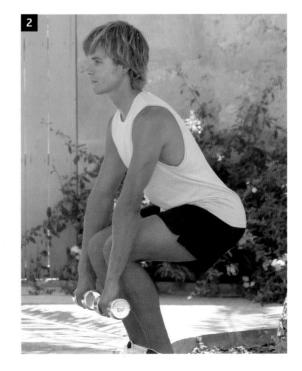

Squat and press with dumbbells 2 Sets 15 Reps

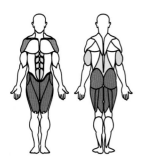

The muscles being worked are the quads, hamstrings, glutes, deltoids, and triceps. Try not to swing the weights or use any momentum. Keep the form of the exercise strict and under control. Squat and press!

1 From a standing position, grasp a set of dumbbells. Hold them on either side of your collarbone, with the palms of your hands facing away from you. Activate your core muscles.

2 With your stance at shoulder width, squat down bending at the knees. Press upward with the glutes, and while doing so, press the dumbbells above the head. Lower the dumbbells under control.

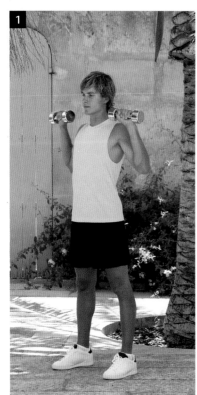

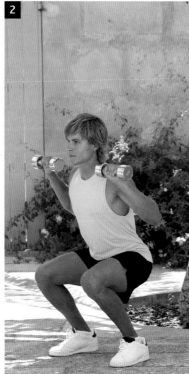

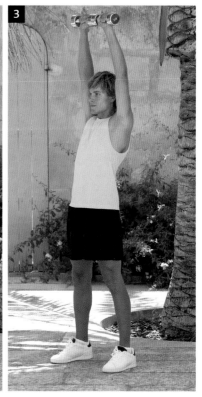

One-arm row with dumbbells 2 Sets 12 Reps

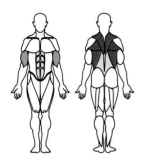

The muscles being worked are the latissimus dorsi, rhomboids, trapezius, and biceps. Keep your back straight throughout this exercise.

1 With your stance at hip width, grasp the dumbbells, palms facing each other. Lean forward bending at the knees and hips, ensuring your back is straight and arms at length.

2 Squeeze the muscles in the upper back as you draw one dumbbell in toward you. Keep your elbow in and back. Lower under control and repeat with the other dumbbell, alternating arms.

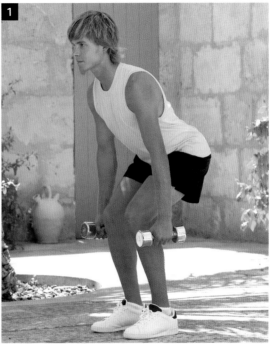

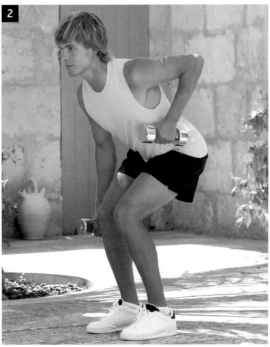

Two-arm bench press with barbell 2 Sets 12 Reps

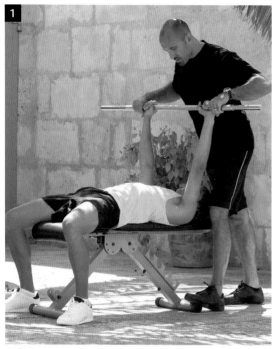

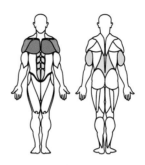

The muscles being worked are the pectorals, deltoids, and triceps. It's amazing what can be achieved when linking the mind and muscle together. Imagine the chest working. Feel! Control! Resist!

1 Lie on a flat-position bench and grasp a barbell with an overhand grip, with your hands one and a half times shoulder-width apart. Keep your arms straight but not locked. Activate your core muscles.

2 Lower the resistance under control, so that the bar is in line with your nipples. Press the bar upward to the start position using the chest muscles, as well as the arms.

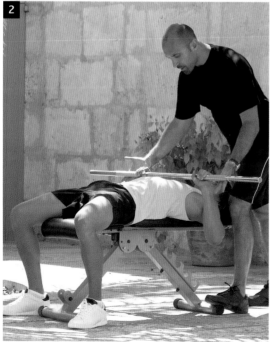

Two-arm standing row with dumbbells 2 Sets 12 Reps

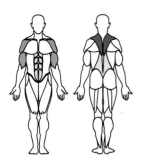

The muscles being worked are the trapezius, deltoids, and biceps. Once the dumbbells are raised, the elbows should be in line with your ears. This is a great exercise for the development of the overall shoulder area.

1 Using a set of dumbbells, arms at length and the palms facing you, place your left leg forward, right leg back. Activate your core muscles.

2 Lead with the elbows and raise the dumbbells toward your chin, stopping at the collarbone. Bend the elbows and contract the deltoids. Lower the weight back to the starting position.

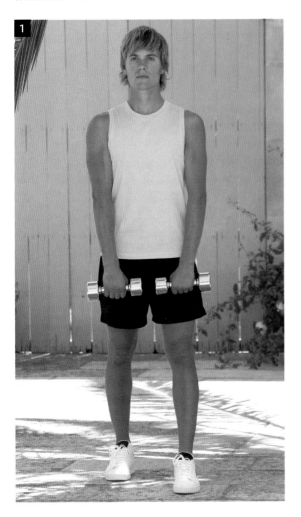

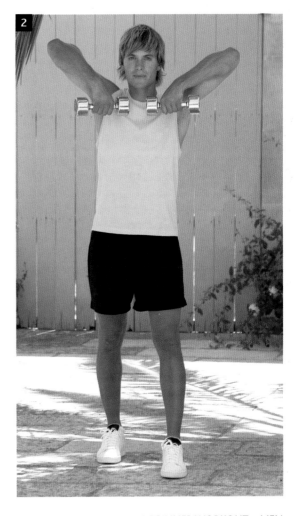

Two-arm standing shoulder press with barbell 2 Sets 12 Reps

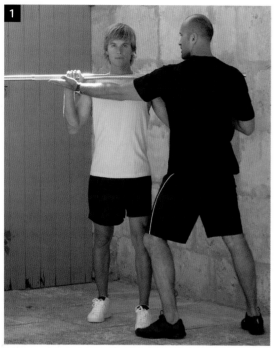

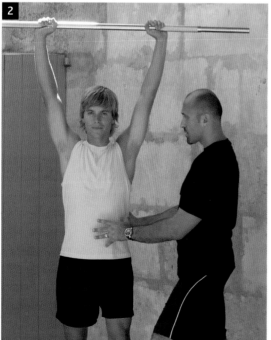

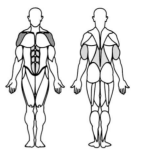

The muscles being worked are the deltoids and triceps. Breathe out on the exertion and keep those arms moving at the correct speed, 2 seconds up, 2 seconds down!

1 Grasp a barbell with your hands on either side of you at shoulder point, palms facing away from you. Stand with one foot in front of the other.

2 Press the barbell above your head until your arms are straight but not locked. Lower the resistance under control back to shoulder point and repeat the movement.

Two-arm lying triceps extension with barbell 2 Sets 12 Reps

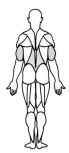

The muscles being worked are the triceps. Try to avoid allowing your elbows to swing out to the sides with this exercise. Initially, practice the execution of the movement before increasing the weight.

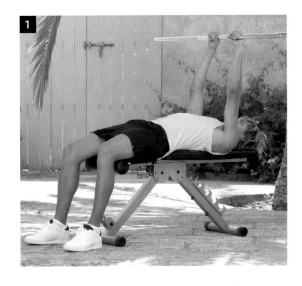

1 Lying on a flat bench, grasp a barbell. Position your hands so that they are two thumb-widths apart. With your palms facing away from you extend your arms. Activate your core muscles.

2 Bend at the elbow joints, keeping your shoulders totally still, and allowing the barbell to go just past your forehead. Press with the triceps back to the start position.

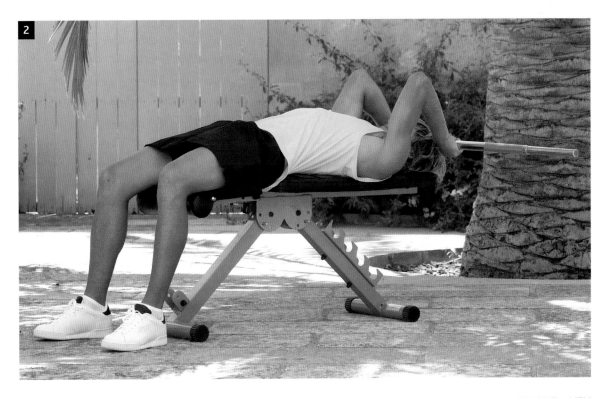

Two-arm standing biceps curl with barbell 2 Sets 12 Reps

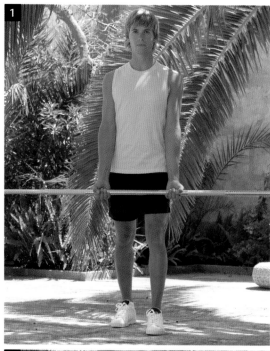

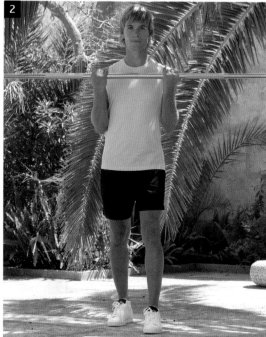

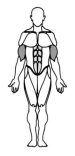

The muscles being worked are the biceps. Flex the biceps at the top of the movement and don't let those muscles rest!

1 From a standing position, left leg forward, right leg back, grasp a barbell, palms facing away from you.

2 With your elbows locked into your sides, curl the barbell up toward your collarbone. Lower the weight under control, keeping your elbows soft.

Oblique twists 2 Sets 12 Reps

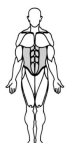

The muscles being worked are the internal and external obliques. This is such a great movement that totally isolates the working area. Make sure to coordinate the movement correctly.

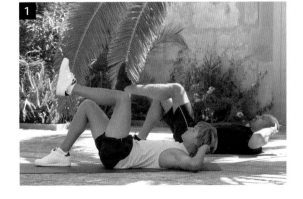

1 Lying on an exercise mat, semiflex the left leg and place your hands behind your head.

2 With your hands supporting the head, rotate your torso bringing your right elbow across your body, allowing the shoulder blade to come off the floor. Bring your left knee toward the elbow allowing the oblique to contract. Now change sides.

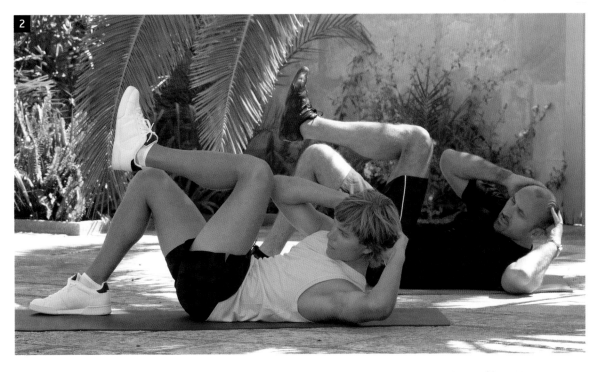

Ball crunches 2 Sets 20 Reps

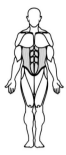

The muscles being worked here are the rectus abdomen. Small movements are required to keep the abs constantly working. It's surprising how easily you can isolate the abdomen. Feel the burn!

1 Lying on an exercise mat, place your bent legs on either side of the stability ball, your hands behind your head, and raise your shoulder blades off the floor.

2 Keeping the ball still, raise your shoulders off the ground and crunch upward allowing the abdomen to contract. Breathe out. Return to the start position.

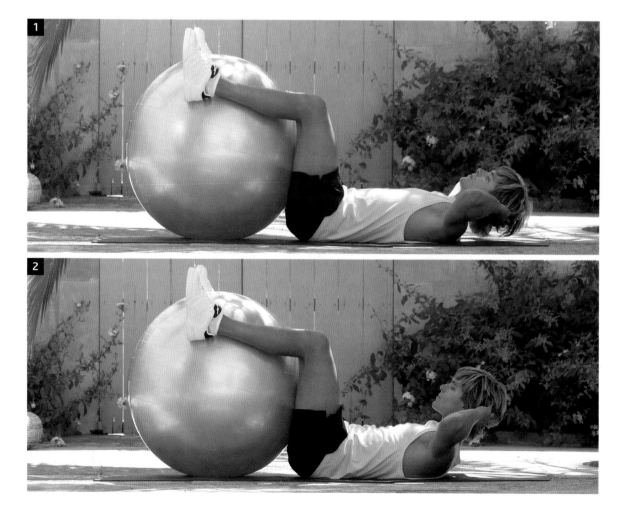

The plank 2 Sets 20 Reps

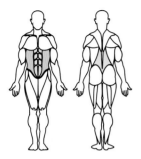

The entire core area is being worked on here. Try to breathe normally when doing this challenging exercise and focus on tightening the relevant muscles.

1 Activate your core muscles, drawing your navel to your spine. Resting on your forearms and toes, hold your body up. Keep your elbows under your shoulder blades with your forearms facing forward.

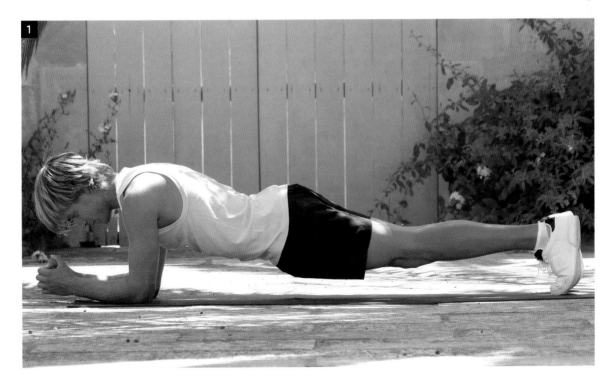

3 Intermediate workout for women

Now you have just 30 seconds rest between exercises. Keep to the same speed of repetitions, and think about the muscles working!

Walking lunges with dumbbells 2 Sets 20 Reps

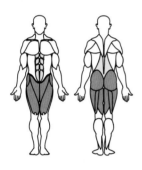

The muscles being worked are the quads, hamstrings, and glutes. Pay close attention to your balance. Link mind and muscle while performing the movement.

1 From a standing position, grasp a set of dumbbells, palms facing each other, and activate your core muscles. Lunge forward keeping your back straight and arms at length.

2 Bend at your hips, knees, and ankles, so that the rear leg is one inch from the ground.

3 Push upward, and immediately step forward with the other leg and repeat the sequence.

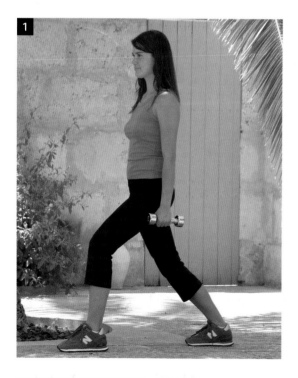

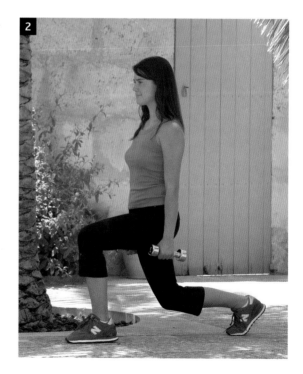

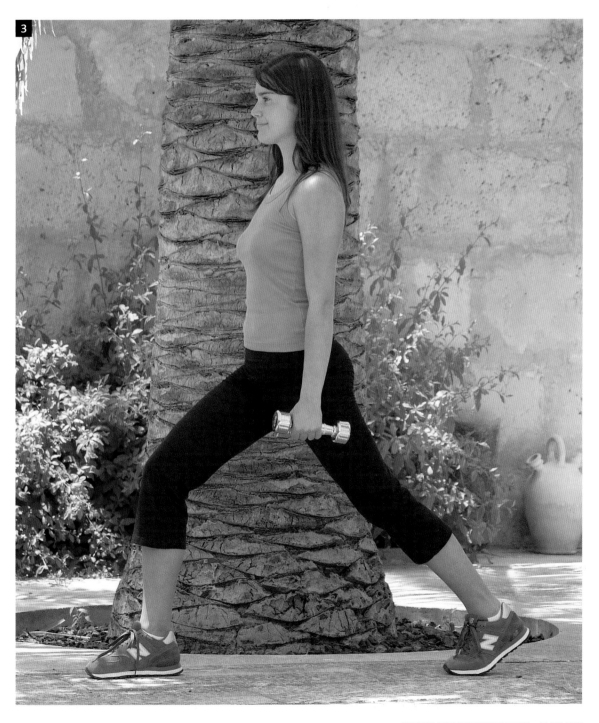

3

Ball squats 2 Sets 25 Reps

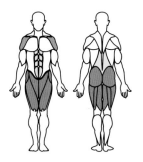

The muscles being worked are the quads, hamstrings, glutes, adductors, and deltoids. This is a total body exercise with emphasis on your inner thighs. Keep your body moving throughout this exercise, and push through your heels.

1 With your feet wide apart, make sure that your knees and toes are in line, and your toes are pointing outward at 11 and 1 o'clock. Using a medicine ball or soccer ball, squat down under control, so that your thighs are parallel to the floor. Activate your core muscles.

2 Throw the ball up, allowing you enough time to stand up tall, and then to squat down to the start position.

3 Catch the ball at the lowest point, and repeat the sequence again.

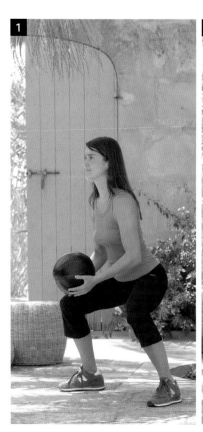

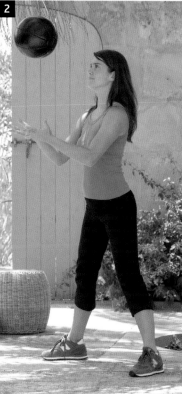

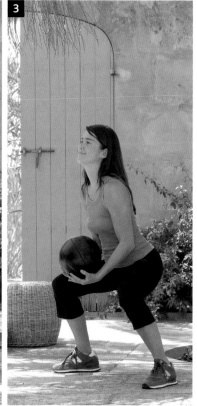

Ball dead-lifts 2 Sets 25 Reps

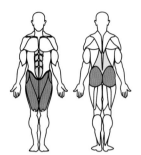

The muscles being worked are the quads and glutes. This is a great overall body exercise. Keep the form of the exercise smooth and perfect.

1 Grasp a medicine ball or soccer ball and make sure your hips, knees, and toes are in line with your stance at hip width. Activate your core muscles.

2 Lower yourself down, keeping your back and arms straight, and place the ball on the ground. Now push through your glutes and return to the start position. Don't let your knees travel past your toes. Repeat the sequence.

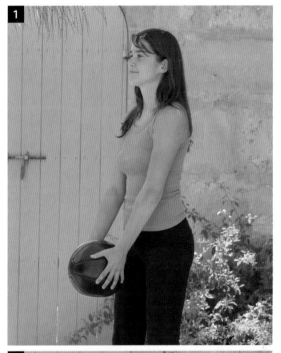

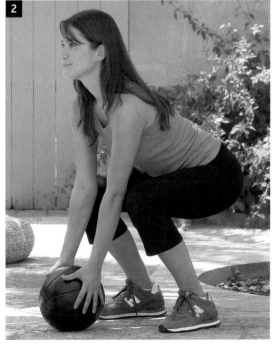

Stiff-legged dead-lift with dumbbells 2 Sets 25 Reps

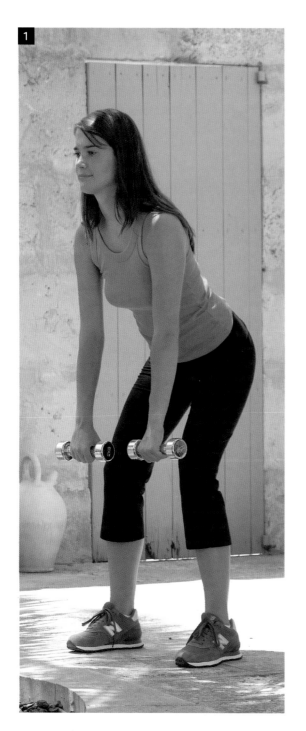

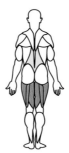

The muscles being worked are the hamstrings. Focus on the working muscles! Remember to keep the speed of the movement 2 seconds up, 2 seconds down.

1 Make sure your hips, knees, and toes are in line. Move forward from your torso so that the dumbbells are at knee level and your back is straight.

2 Perform small micro-movements, up and down, from the torso, keeping your back and arms straight.

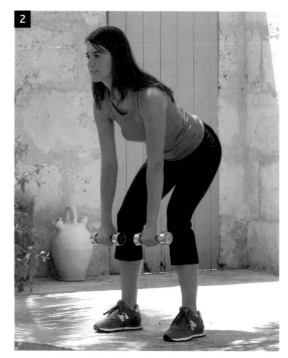

Two-arm row with dumbbells 2 Sets 12 Reps

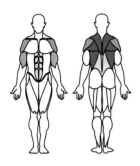

The muscles being worked are the latissimus dorsi, rhomboids, trapezius, deltoids, and biceps. This exercise is great for toning the main back and shoulder muscles.

1 From a narrow stance, grasp the dumbbells, palms facing each other. Lean forward. Keep your back straight and arms at length.

2 Squeeze your shoulder blades together and draw the dumbbells in toward your chest. Keep your elbows in and back. Lower under control and repeat.

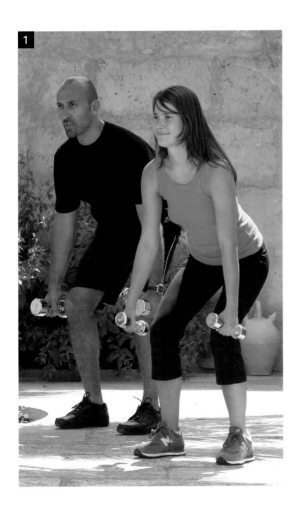

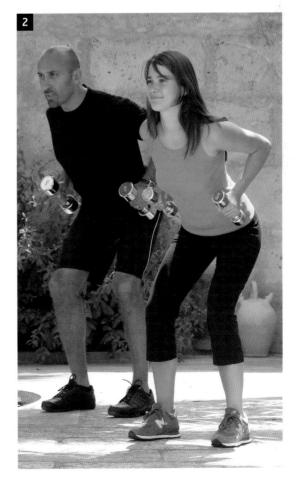

Rear shoulder flys with dumbbells 2 Sets 12-15 Reps

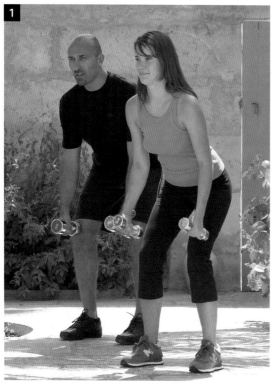

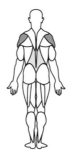

The muscles being worked are the rear deltoids. This is a fabulous exercise that works the upper back, with major emphasis on the rear shoulders. Avoid momentum and keep the back nicely angled at 70 degrees to the floor.

1 From a narrow stance grasp the dumbbells, palms facing each other. Lean forward. Keep your arms straight with your elbows soft and your back straight. Activate your core muscles.

2 Perform a flying action with your arms, keeping the palms of your hands facing the ground. Make sure to keep the elbows soft, and raise the arms up to shoulder point. Lower the weight under control, and repeat the sequence.

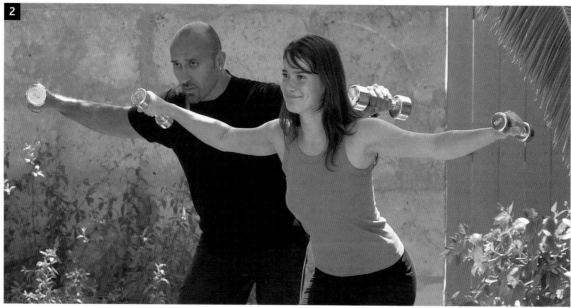

Chest flys with dumbbells 2 Sets 12 Reps

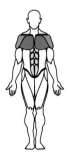

The muscles being worked are the pectorals and anterior deltoids. This exercise isolates the muscles in the chest and the front shoulders. Squeeze your pectorals at the highest point at the start of the exercise for greater condition.

1 Lying on a mat, take a neutral grip on the dumbbells, palms facing each other, and raise your arms with your elbows slightly flexed. Activate your core muscles.

2 Lower the weight under control and contract your chest. Raise the dumbbells to the starting position.

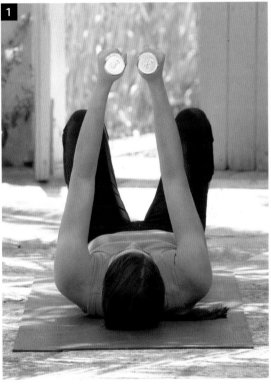

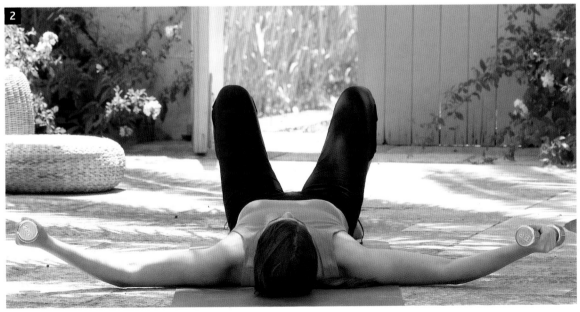

Chest press on stability ball with dumbbells 2 Sets 12 Reps

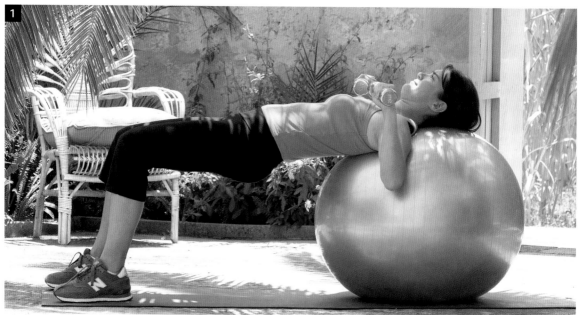

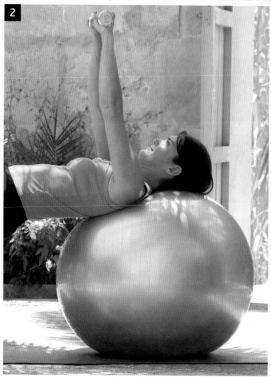

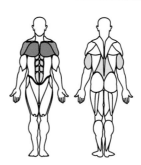

This is a compound exercise that works your chest, anterior deltoids, and triceps. Maintain good balance with this exercise. Press with your chest, and not with your arms. Try to link your mind with your muscles.

1 Begin with your head and shoulders on the stability ball. Try to keep your hips parallel to the ground and maintain a stable posture. Activate your core muscles.

2 Press the dumbbells up with your elbows to the side, until your arms are extended. Repeat the sequence.

Shoulder press on stability ball with dumbbells 2 Sets 12 Reps

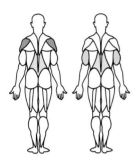

The muscles being worked are the deltoids and triceps. Try not to allow your body to lean back or rock during this exercise. Feel the muscles burn!

1 Sit tall on the ball, maintaining a stable posture. Start by holding the dumbbells on either side of your collarbone, palms facing out. Activate your core muscles.

2 Press one dumbbell overhead with the arm fully extended but not locked. Lower under control. Alternate with the other arm.

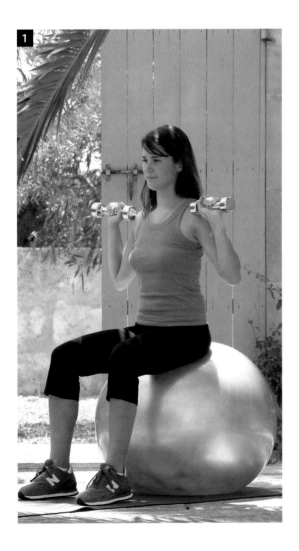

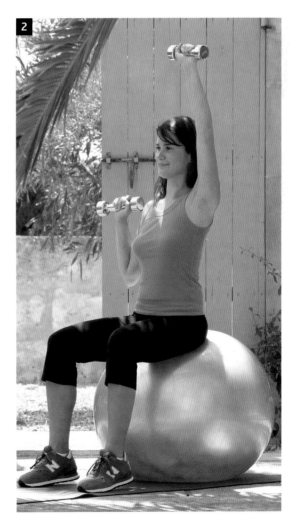

Unilateral dumbbell triceps extension on stability ball 2 Sets 12 Reps

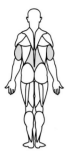

Try to avoid letting your elbows sway to the side. Press only with your triceps and avoid any other muscles coming into play. You think it's that easy?

1 Sit on a stability ball maintaining a stable posture. Feet hip-width apart, activate your core muscles. Fold one arm across your abdomen.

2 With the other arm grasping a dumbbell, bend at the elbow and let the forearm lower the dumbbell past the head. Return to the start position.

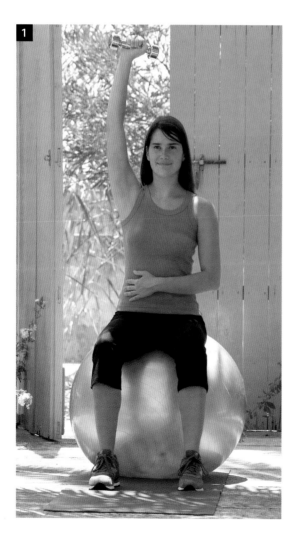

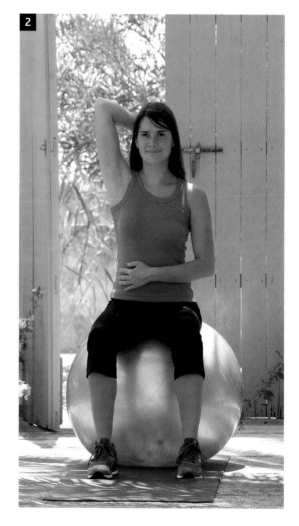

Tricep extension on stability ball with dumbbell 1 Set 12–15 Reps

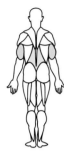

For this exercise you'll need a slightly heavier dumbbell than you've used so far. Remember, 2 seconds up, 2 seconds down.

1 Sit on a stability ball maintaining a stable posture. Feet hip-width apart, activate your core muscles. Now with both arms, grasp a dumbbell and extend your arms.

2 Bend your elbows allowing the dumbbell to fall behind you. Extend to the start position and repeat.

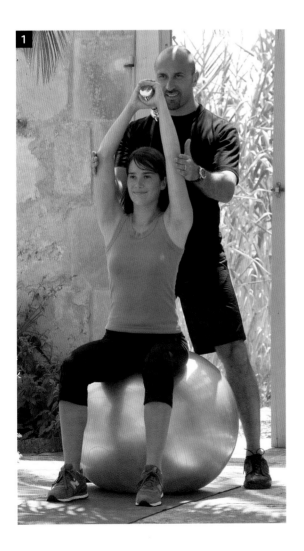

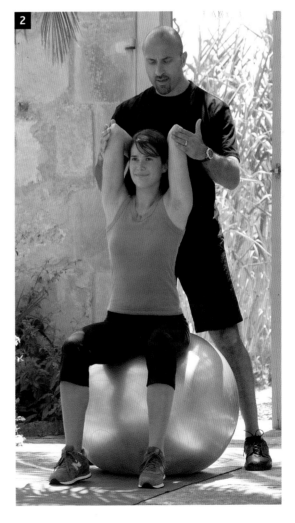

Two-arm biceps curl on stability ball with dumbbells

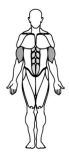

The muscles being worked are the biceps. Stay upright while performing the full range of joint movements. Work those biceps!

1 Sit on a stability ball maintaining a stable posture and keep the spine upright. Grasping the dumbbells with palms facing away from you, pull both elbows in toward the sides of the body and perform a biceps curl.

2 As the curl reaches its peak, stop and return to the start position.

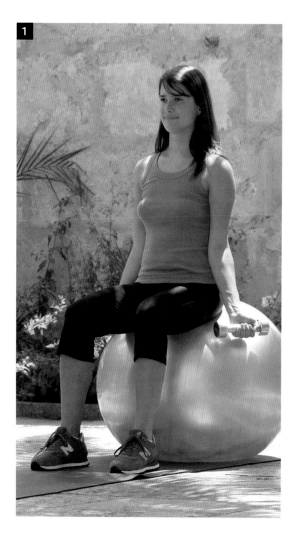

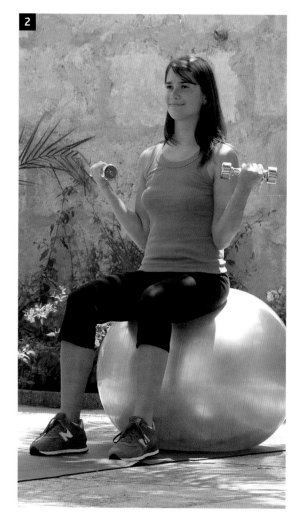

3 Once you've done 6 repetitions of the previous exercise, change the position of the hands, so that the palms are facing each other.

4 Curl again for 6 repetitions and return to the start position.

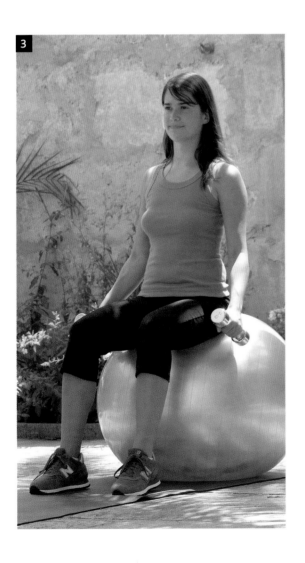

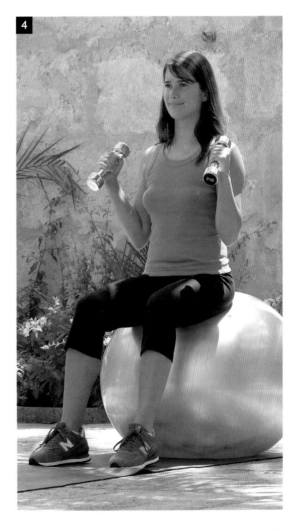

Oblique waist workers 2 Sets 20 Reps

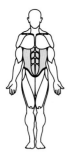

The muscles being worked are the obliques and rectus abdomen. This is a fantastic exercise for your obliques and abdomen. Don't arch your back and concentrate on the movement. Go for it!

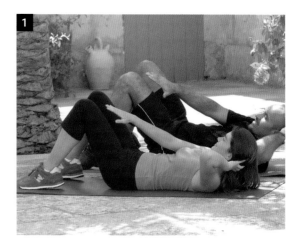

1 Lying on a mat, place one hand behind your head and raise your heels. Activate your core muscles. Draw in your navel to your spine.

2 Keep one arm straight and across the body just above the opposite knee. Pivot the upper body through the hips gently rotating the arm around the knee. Raise your side shoulder blade off the floor.

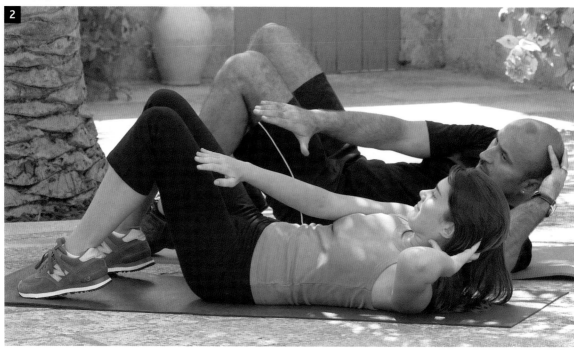

Abdominal rockers 2 Sets 20 Reps

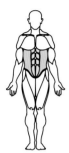

The muscles being worked are the rectus abdomen. Smooth, micro-movements are required, pulling from the abdomen. Don't underestimate this exercise. It starts off easily and gradually begins to burn!

1 Lying on a flat bench, raise your legs. With your knees slightly bent and legs at 90 degrees, position your feet so they are facing toward the ceiling. Keep your legs slightly bent and place your arms behind your head. Activate your core muscles.

2 With your hands behind your head and ideally grasping a bench, move from the hips keeping your lower back flat. Squeeze, control, contract. Come on!

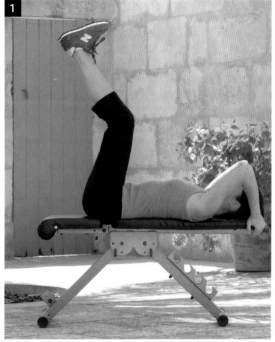

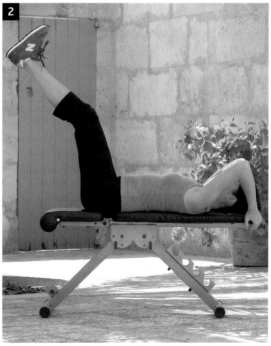

Ball circuit 2 Sets 20 Reps

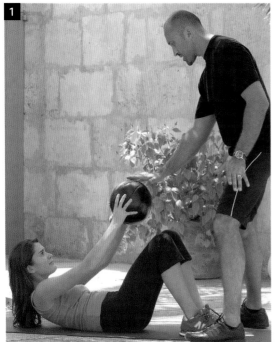

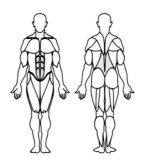

The muscles being worked are the entire core area. Avoid arching your back and using momentum. Make sure to breathe out always on the exertion. This is a great exercise to perform with a partner. Use a medicine ball or a soccer ball.

1 Lying on a mat grasp a medicine ball. Activate your core muscles. With your feet flat on the floor, perform a normal sit-up.

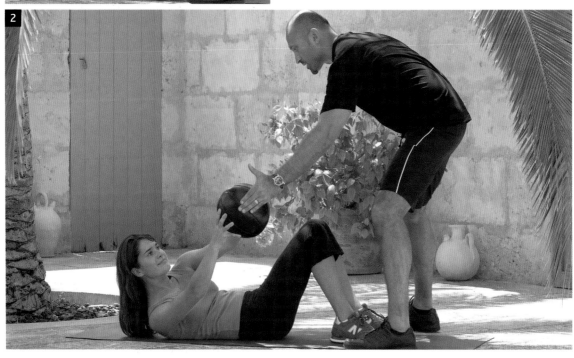

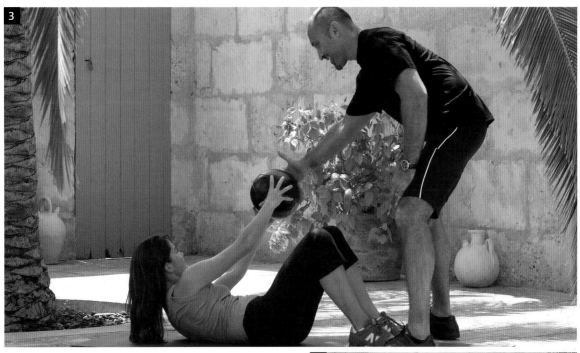

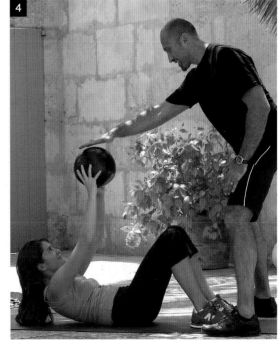

2 Now raise your shoulder blade and push to one side, still holding the ball outstretched in your hands.

3 Return to the start position and now push to the other side again, still holding the ball.

4 Return to the start position and now reach upward. Repeat the circuit.

4

Intermediate workout for men

Now with only 30 seconds rest between sets, we've just moved up a level! Think about the muscles working!

Side squats with dumbbells 2 Sets 12–15 Reps

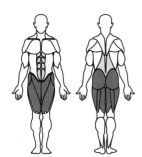

The muscles being worked are the quads, hamstrings, glutes, and adductors. Keep your thighs parallel to the floor when squatting. Don't use momentum and breathe out when you exert!

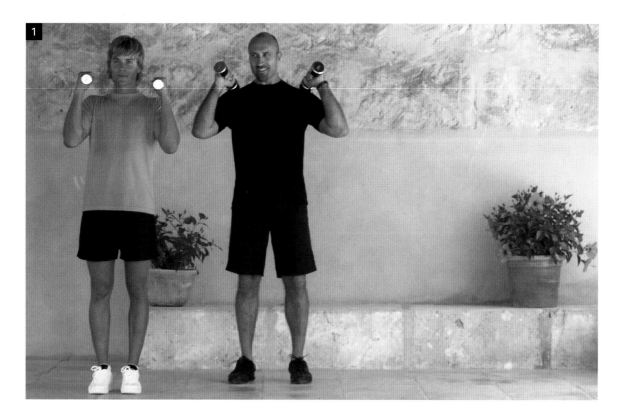

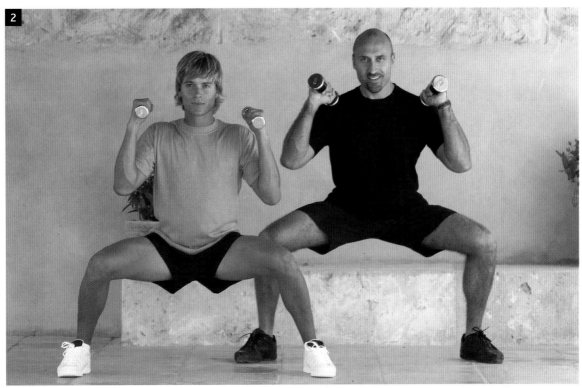

1 With a hip-width stance, grasp the dumbbells on either side of your collarbone. Activate your core muscles, drawing your navel to your spine.

2 With your right leg, step sideways into a squat, feet past shoulder width, hips, knees, and toes in line. Under control, bend your knees and lower yourself toward the ground, keeping your back totally straight.

3 Press from the glutes, moving your left leg inward as you stand up. Move smoothly and repeat the movement.

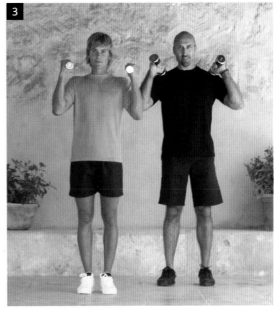

Knee dips 2 Sets 12–15 Reps

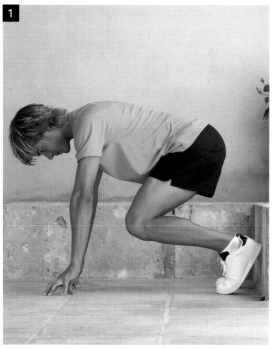

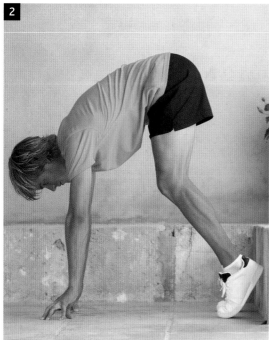

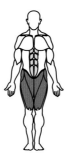

The muscles being worked here are the quads. This exercise totally isolates your front thighs. Try not to allow your knees to go too low during this exercise, and avoid locking the knees out at the high point. Keep your body moving.

1 Get yourself into a sprinter's position with your heels against a wall and your toes on the floor. Activate your core muscles. Slowly lower both knees until they reach just below your elbows.

2 Push both legs up and back until extended. Under control, return to the start position. Try to keep your legs moving throughout this exercise. Stabilize your upper body.

Barbell dead-lift to shoulder shrug to calf raise   2 Sets 12–15 Reps

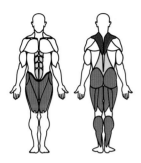

The muscles being worked are the gastrocnemius, quads, glutes, and trapezius. This is a great total-body exercise. Initially, break the movement into three individual lifts. As your strength and technique improves, the movement will become fluent.

1 Stand with your feet hip-width apart, drawing your navel into your spine. Make sure your hips, knees, and toes are in line. Grasp the barbell in both hands holding it with your arms straight.

2 Activate your core muscles and lower yourself down into a dead-lift position, keeping your back straight. Push through your glutes, keeping your head up. Go back to the start position.

3 Immediately perform a shrugging action, drawing your shoulders upward. Raise yourself and move up onto your toes, lifting the heels off the ground to perform a calf raise. Return to the start position and repeat.

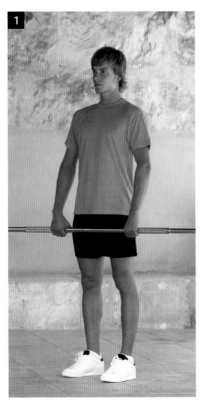

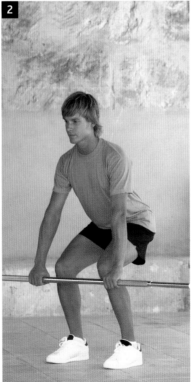

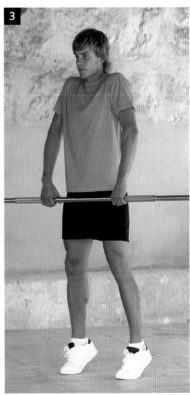

Two-arm reverse row with barbell 2 Sets 12 Reps

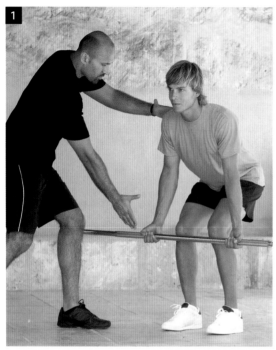

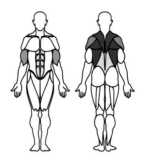

The muscles being worked are the latissimus dorsi, rhomboids, trapezius, lower lumbar, rear deltoid, and biceps. This exercise works the whole back area.

This is, by far, one of the best exercises for your back for strength and condition.

1 Stand with your feet hip-width apart. Grasp the bar with your palms facing away from your body. Bend the upper torso to a 70-degree angle. Keep your back straight throughout the full range of movement, and your hips, knees, and toes in line. Activate your core muscles.

2 Keeping the elbows angled toward your sides, squeeze your shoulder blades together, as the bar reaches chest level. Try to keep the arms moving. Return to the start position.

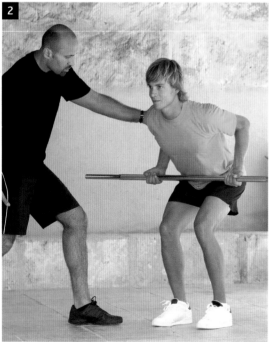

SUPERSET:
Incline unilateral chest press with dumbbells 2 Sets 12 reps

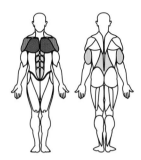

The muscles being worked are the pectorals, deltoids, and triceps. Focus on the upper chest and work on your mind and muscle connection.

1 On an incline bench, grasp the dumbbells with your palms facing away from you. Raise your arms so the dumbbells are above your head. Activate your core muscles.

2 Bending one arm, lower the weight down so the dumbbell reaches the outside of the chest. Press upward and repeat the movement. Once the 12 reps have been performed, change arms. To complete the Superset, move straight to step 3 without stopping. (cont. on page 72)

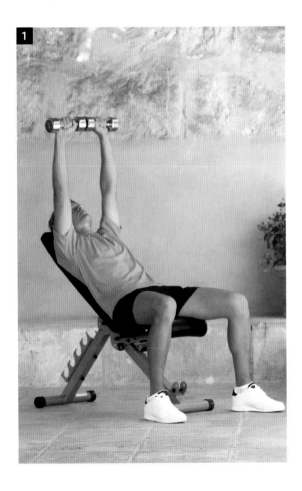

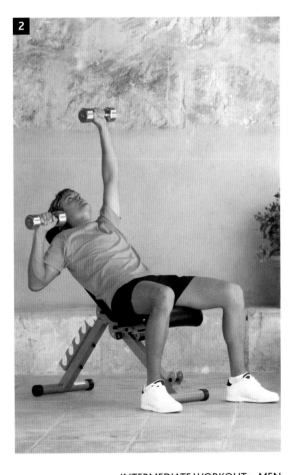

SUPERSET:
Two-arm chest flys with dumbbells 2 Sets 12 Reps

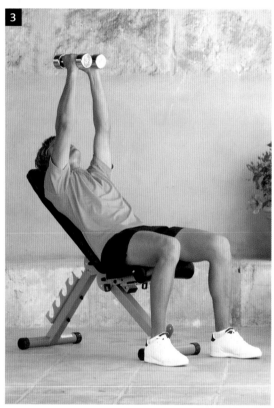

(cont. from page 71)

3 Extend your arms with the elbows slightly flexed and in line with your upper chest. Now hold the dumbbells with your palms facing inward. Activate your core muscles.

4 Lower the weights with both your arms under control, so that the dumbbells are in line with your ears. Contract the chest muscles and raise your arms to the start position. Now move back to step 1 and repeat the sequence.

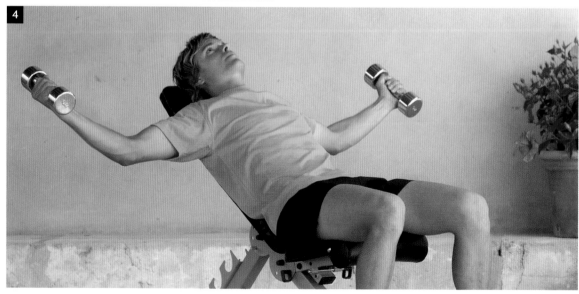

Two-arm standing lateral raise with dumbbell 2 Sets 12 Reps

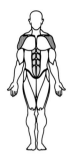

The muscles being worked are the medial deltoids. Try not to lift your elbows above shoulder height. Concentrate on your muscles and your movement.

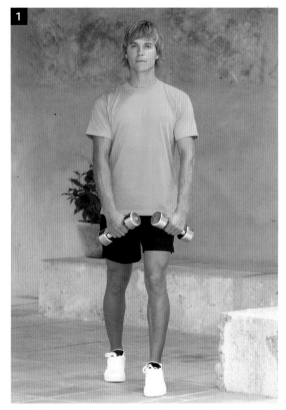

1 From a standing position grasp a set of dumbbells. Put one leg in front of the other. Grasp the dumbbells with your palms facing you. Activate your core muscles.

2 Lift both arms laterally to shoulder height, keeping the elbows soft and the palms facing the floor. Return to the start position.

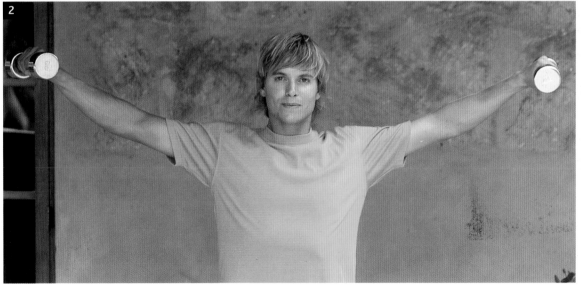

Shoulder press on stability ball with dumbbells 2 Sets 12 Reps

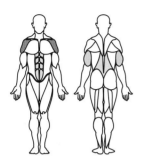

The muscles being worked on are the anterior deltoids and triceps. Try pressing both dumbbells upward and rotating halfway through the movement, so that the dumbbells are facing away from you. This becomes a two-arm dumbbell Arnold Press.

1 Sit upright on a stability ball and maintain stable posture. Keep your back straight throughout the exercise. Hold the dumbbells either side of your collarbone, palms facing each other.

2 Press both dumbbells upward until the arms are extended but not fully locked. Lower under control and repeat.

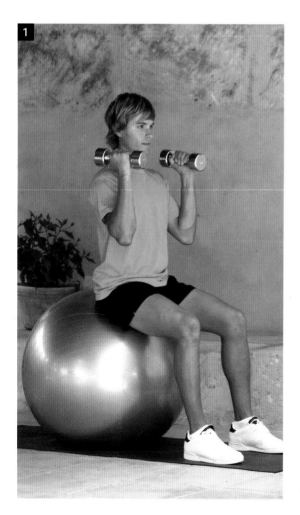

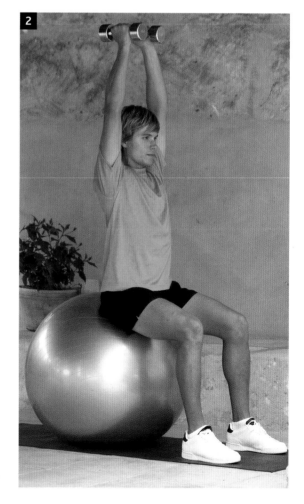

Two-arm overhead tricep extension 2 Sets 12 Reps

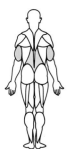

The muscles being worked are the triceps. Try to avoid allowing your elbows to sway to the side, and press upward with the working triceps. This is one of the best exercises for your triceps, ever!

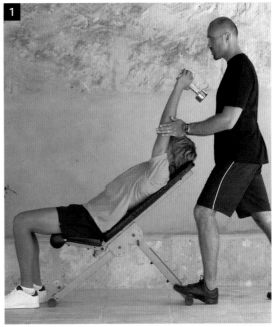

1 Lie back on the bench and grasp the dumbbells, raising your arms so that your elbows cover your ears.

2 Bend only at the elbows, let the forearms lower the dumbbell to the outside of the ear.

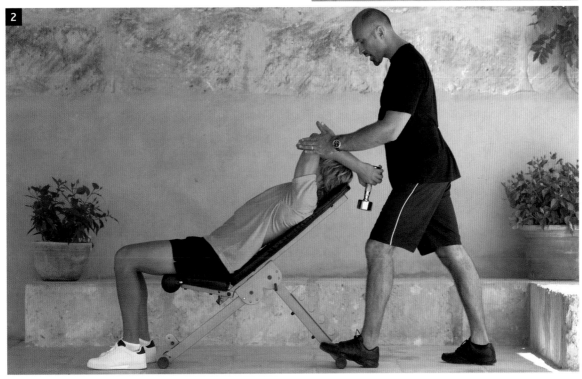

Incline biceps curl with dumbbells 2 Sets 12 Reps

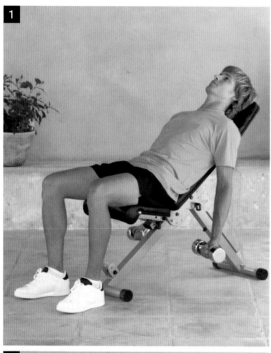

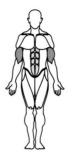

The muscles being worked are the biceps. Try to avoid any movement of your upper arm. Squeeze your bicep at the highest point and feel the contraction.

1 While seated in an incline position grasp the dumbbells with your palms facing out away from you. Lower your arms, keeping your elbows soft. Activate your core muscles.

2 Pull both elbows in toward the side of your body and perform a bicep curl. As the curl reaches its peak, stop and return to the start position.

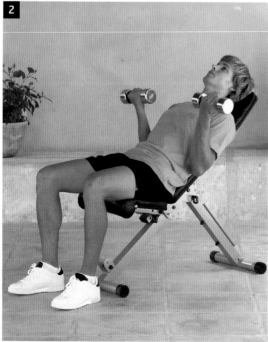

Micro abdominal crunches 2 Sets 20 Reps

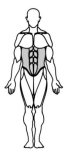

The muscles being worked are the rectus abdomen. Keep your hands uncrossed, and avoid pulling your neck muscles. Work your abs! Pump it!

1 Lie on a mat, placing your hands behind your head for support and raise your heels. Activate your core muscles, drawing your navel to your spine. Keep your shoulder blades off the floor throughout the range of movement and keep the abs contracted.

2 Curl your upper torso up while pressing your lower back into the mat. Repeat the sequence. The movement should be continuous.

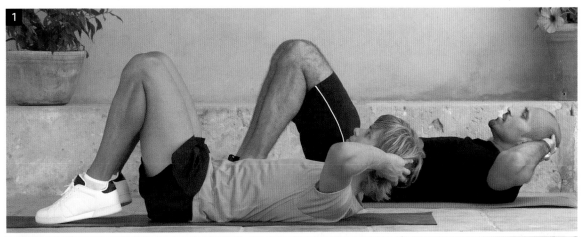

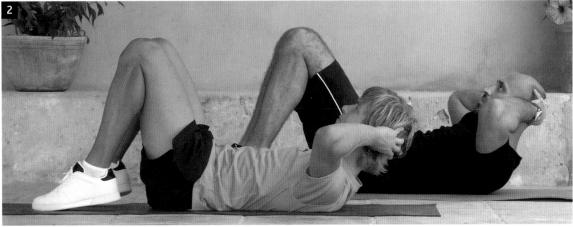

Ball obliques 2 Sets 20 Reps

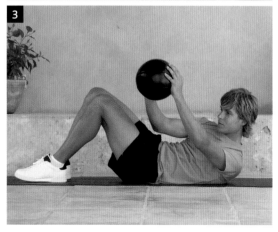

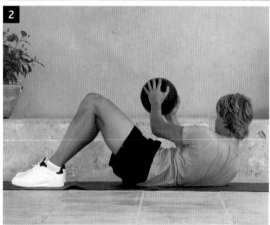

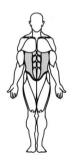

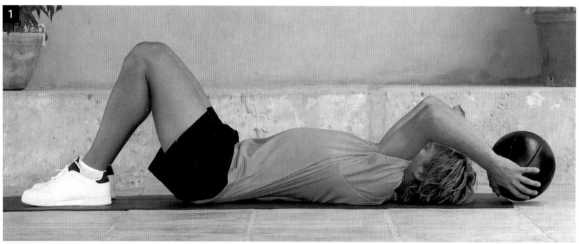

The muscles being worked are the obliques. Don't use momentum! Control the movement and grind out those reps!

1 Lie on a mat. With a medicine ball or soccer ball, start with the ball behind your head, and your lower back pressed against the floor. Activate your core muscles.

2 Lift with the abdomen and raise the ball over your head in one direction.

3 Lower slowly and change the direction.

Lying reverse crunches 1 Set 15–20 Reps

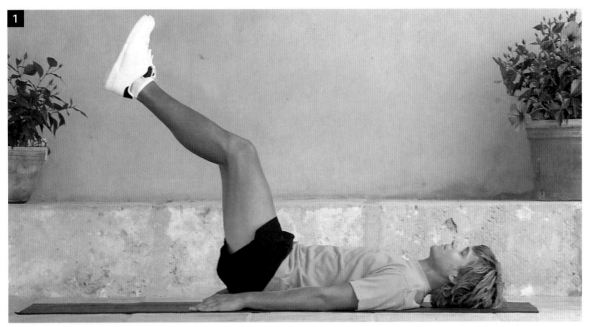

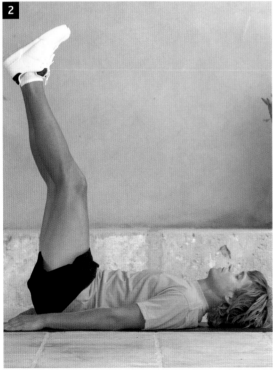

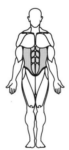

The muscle being worked is the rectus abdomen. Avoid arching your back. If this occurs, your legs have gone too far. Listen to your body and feel the muscle work.

1 Lying on the floor, place your hands on either side of your hips with your legs up. Activate your core muscles.

2 Move from your hips, allowing the legs to come to you, pointing your feet toward the ceiling. Return to the start position. Slow movements are required, squeezing the abs. Keep your lower back on the floor. (cont. on page 80)

Lying reverse crunches with stability ball 1 Set 15–20 Reps

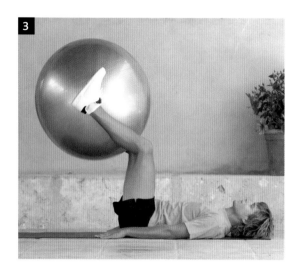

(cont. from page 79)

3 Now grasp a stability ball, with your feet on either side. Repeat the same movement.

4 Come on, work those abs!

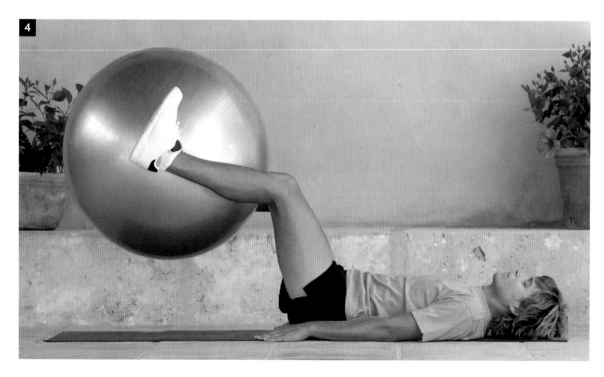

The plank   2 Sets 15–30 Seconds

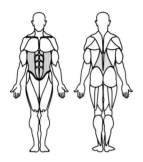

For core stabilization, aim to keep a straight line throughout your legs and spine. Feel your core muscles tighten. Pull in and breathe normally.

1 Resting on your forearms and toes, hold your body up, keep your elbows under your shoulder blades with your forearms facing forward. Activate your core muscles.

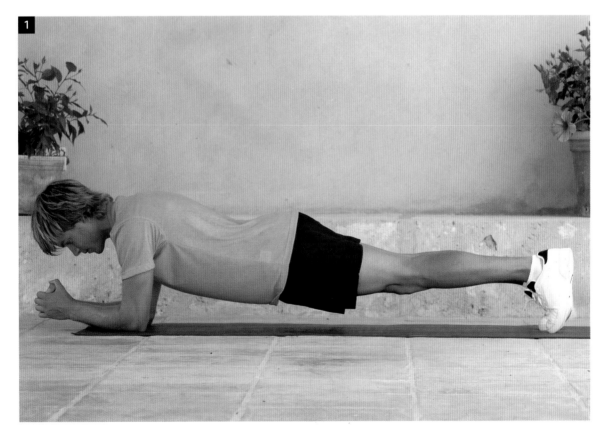

5 Advanced workout for women

Now we're down to 20 seconds rest. Focus on your breathing and work with me!

Concentrated lunges with dumbbells 2 Sets 15 Reps

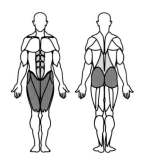

The muscles being worked are the quads and glutes. This is a good exercise for the front of your thighs. Keep your back straight, and allow the muscles to work.

1 Standing on an exercise mat, grasp a set of dumbbells. Position your body so that your left leg is forward, your right leg back, two times shoulder-width apart. Activate your core muscles.

2 Bend at the hip, knee, and ankle, so your bent leg is close to the floor. Push through the front thigh and glutes, and return to the start position. Repeat with the opposite leg.

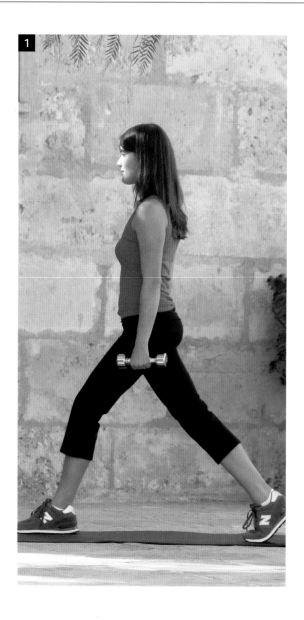

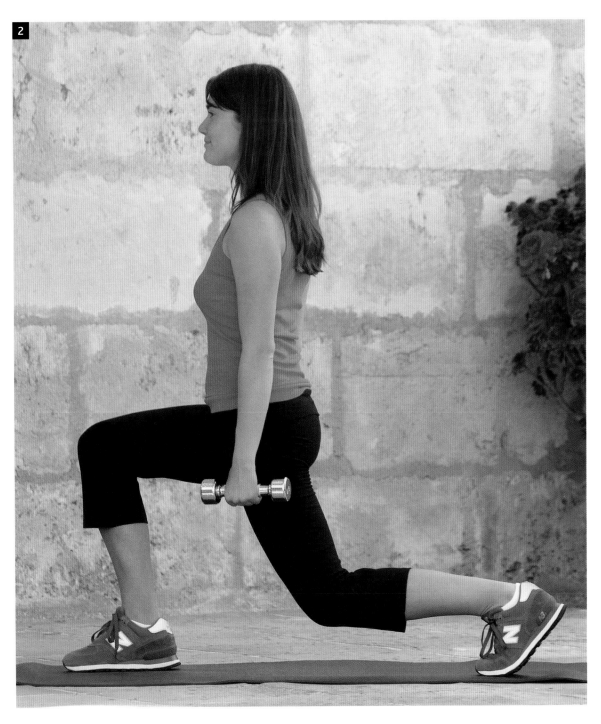

2

Partial hip abduction 2 Sets 21 Reps

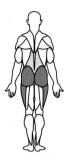

The muscles being worked are the outer thigh abductors and glutes. This exercise isolates the outer thigh muscles, and also causes the glutes to contract. Break the movement down into three and get ready for the burn!

1 Lying on your side, position one leg over the other, bending the lower leg. Do not point your toes. Lift the higher leg so that it is in line with the hip, and return to the start position, bringing the leg down to the floor. Perform 7 reps.

2 Now do the second stage of the movement. Starting with the top leg in line with the hip, lift upward, so that the leg is now slightly above shoulder point. Lower the leg under control until it is in line with the hip. Perform 7 reps.

3 Now perform 7 full-range movements, from the leg's lowest point to its highest. Change sides and repeat the movement.

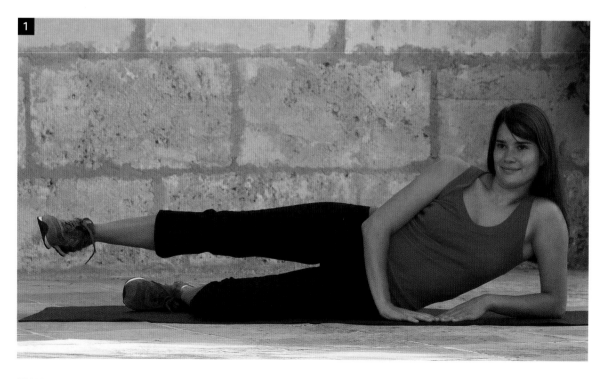

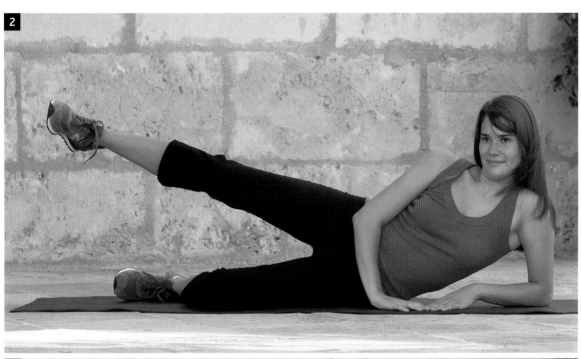

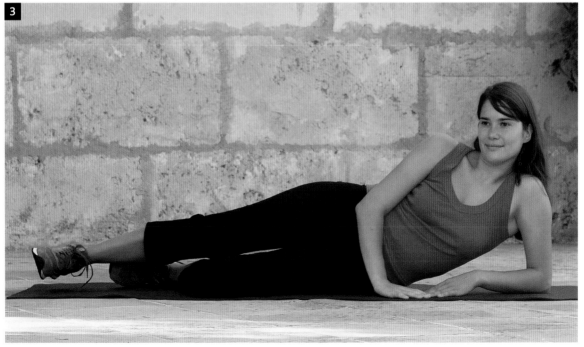

One-legged squat with stability ball 2 Sets 15 Reps

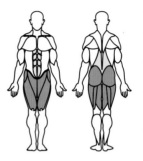

The muscles being worked are the glutes, hamstrings, quads, and the inner thigh adductors. Squeeze the glutes throughout the full range of joint movement, concentrate on balance, and avoid letting your heel come off the floor.

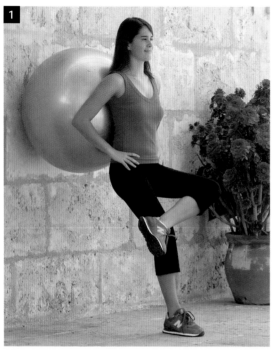

1 Place the stability ball behind you against a wall, level with your lower back. Walk your feet away until you're gently leaning into the ball. Maintain stable posture while bending one leg; place the foot of the bent leg just above the knee. Activate your core muscles.

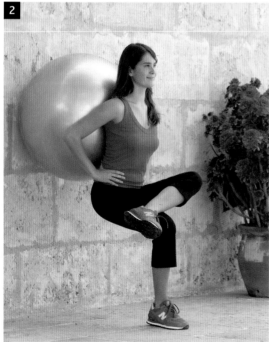

2 Go down into a squat, keeping your back straight, hip, knee, and toes all in line. Return to the start position.

Static ball squats with stability ball and dumbbells 2 Sets 15 Reps

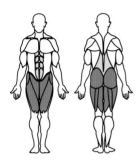

The muscles being worked are the quadriceps, adductors, hamstrings, and glutes. Think about how good your legs are going to look after week 12!

1 With the stability ball behind your back, grasp a set of dumbbells and position them on either side of your collarbone, palms facing each other. Go for a wide stance so that your feet are two times shoulder-width apart.

2 Perform a squat and hold that position for five seconds. Return to start position.

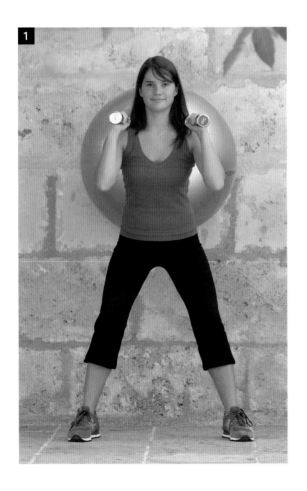

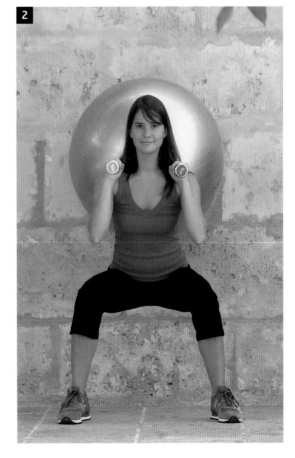

Pullover with medicine ball 2 Sets 12 Reps

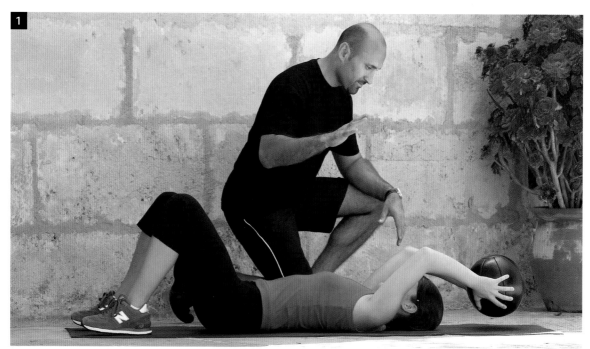

The muscles being worked are the latissimus dorsi and serratus anterior. This is a great exercise for tightening the armpits. Link mind and muscle together, and focus on your back pulling the resistance.

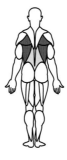

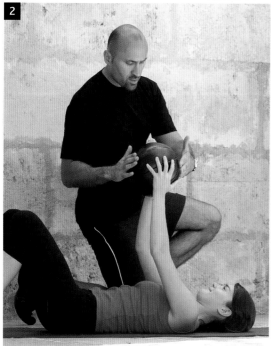

1 Grasping a medicine ball or football, lie down on an exercise mat with your knees bent and feet flat. Hold the ball behind you just off the floor, with your elbows bent. Activate your core muscles.

2 Pull the ball over your head so that it is in line with your chest. Return to the start.

Cobra with dumbbells 2 Sets 15 Reps

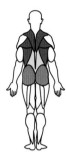

The muscles being worked are the glutes, rhomboids, trapezius, and lower lumbar. This exercise helps your posture and strengthens the muscles in your upper back between your shoulder blades and your neck.

1 Grasp a set of dumbbells and draw in your navel to spine. Stand on one leg, leaning forward and keeping your back straight.

2 With your elbows soft, arch your arms backward, so that the elbows are in line with your hips. Return to the start position.

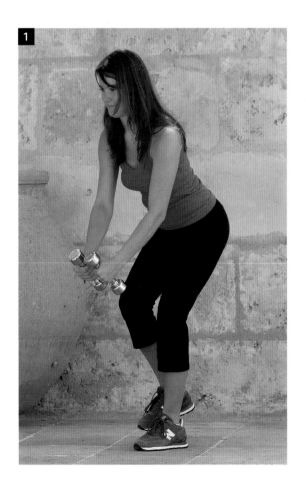

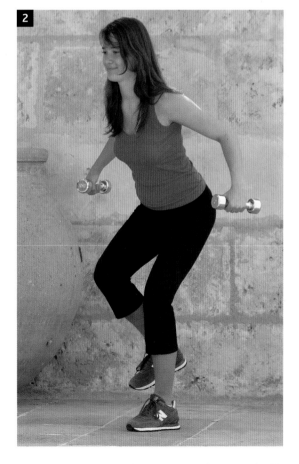

The saw with dumbbells 2 Sets 12 Reps

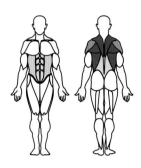

The muscles being worked are the upper back, rear deltoids, and obliques. Squeeze that muscle! Concentrate on the speed of the movement, 2 seconds up, 2 seconds down.

1 From a standing position, grasp a set of dumbbells, palms facing each other, feet hip-width apart. Keeping your back straight, bend forward. Activate your core muscles. Position both your arms in front of you at a 45-degree angle.

2 Pull one arm back in toward you, so that the elbow is past shoulder point.

3 Return to the start position and change arms.

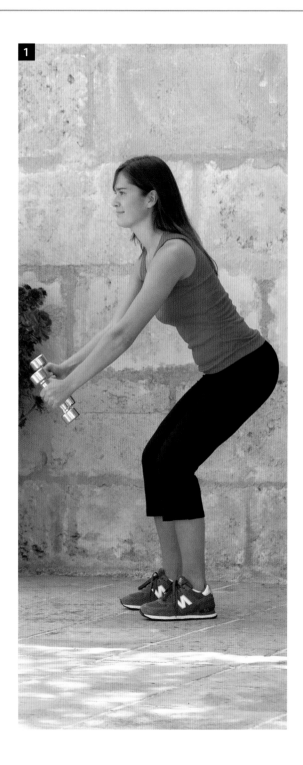

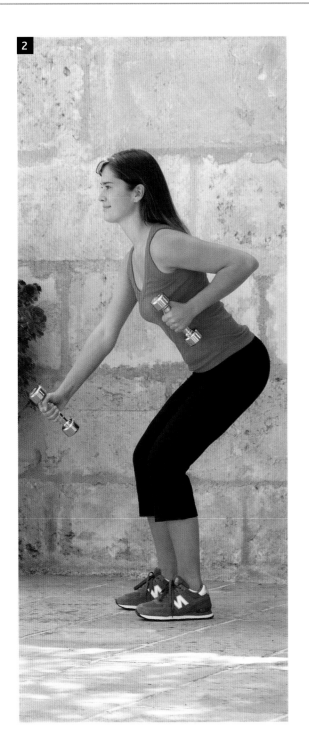

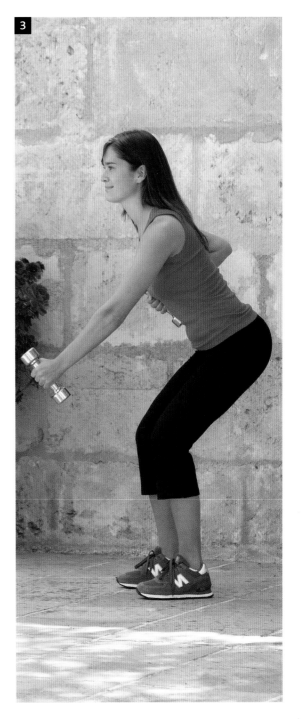

SUPERSET:
Two-arm incline press with barbell 1 Set 12 Reps

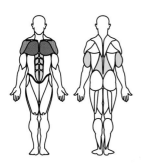

The muscles being worked are the pecs, deltoids, and triceps. Don't waste any time with rest periods. Try and move directly from one exercise to the next, allowing your chest, shoulders, and arms to overload.

1 Lying on a 45-degree incline bench, grasp a barbell on either side of shoulder point, in line with your chin, but not touching your chest, palms facing away from you.

2 Push upward, keeping your arms straight but not locked. Under control, return to the start position and repeat.

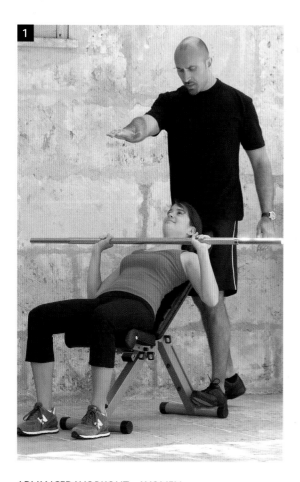

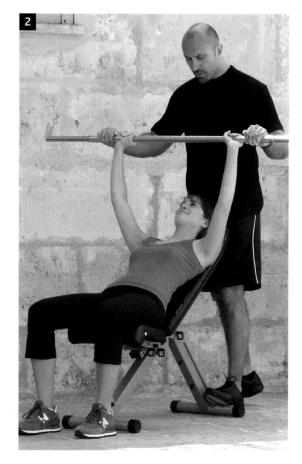

SUPERSET:
Box push-ups 1 Set 12 Reps

Move directly onto the box push-ups.

3 On your hands and knees place your hands on the ground a little wider than shoulder width. Cross your legs behind you.

4 Perform push-ups, in order to keep the body moving. Now return to step 1 and repeat the Superset.

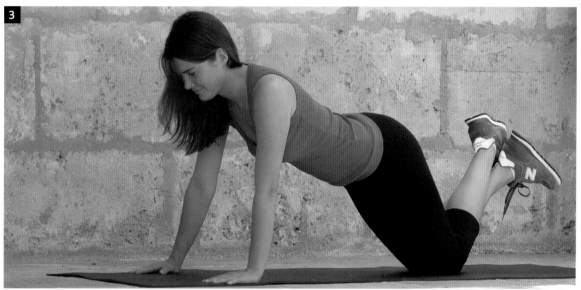

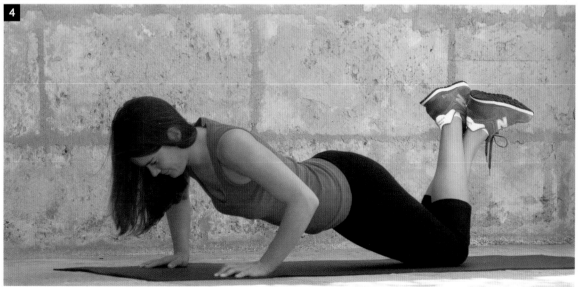

Lateral raise on stability ball 2 Sets 12 Reps

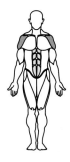

The muscles being worked are the medial deltoids. Keep those arms pumping, don't allow those deltoids to breathe!

1 Sitting on a stability ball, grasp a set of dumbbells, palms facing down. Maintain stable posture and keep your back straight. Activate your core muscles.

2 With your elbows soft, raise both arms out to the sides, until the elbows are in line with your shoulders. Return to the start position.

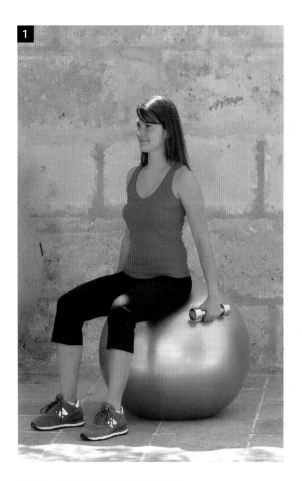

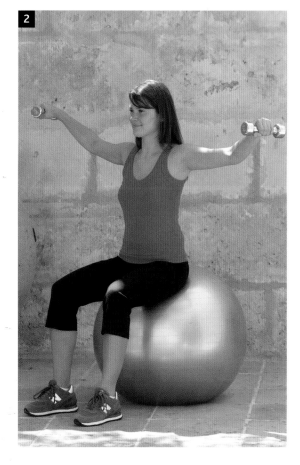

Shoulder press on stability ball with dumbbells 2 Sets 12 Reps

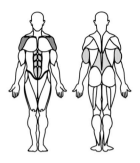

The muscles being worked are the deltoids and triceps. This exercise really isolates the two working muscles. Feel those muscles work, yeah!

1 Sit on a stability ball and maintain a stable posture. Grasping a set of dumbbells, position your hands on either side of your collarbone, palms facing each other. Activate your core muscles, and keep your back straight.

2 With one arm only, press upward, keeping the arm straight, but not locked. Return to the start position and change arms.

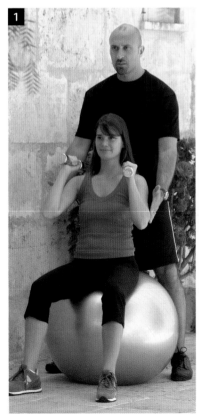

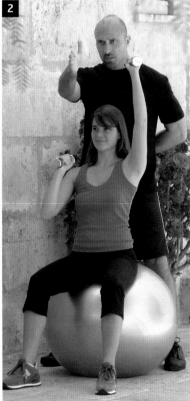

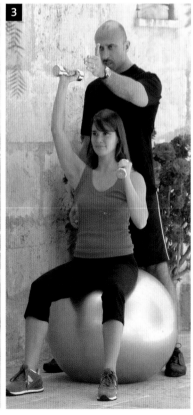

Bench dips 2 Sets 12 Reps

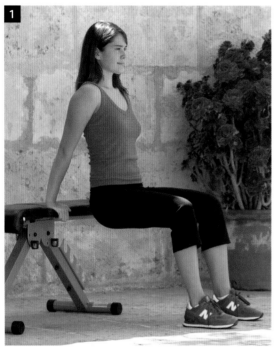

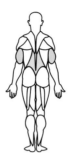

The muscles being worked are the triceps. Avoid letting your shoulders go down too low. Maintain a 90-degree angle at the end position. This is a great exercise for the shape and development of your triceps muscles.

1 With the palms of your hands on the bench behind you, keep your thighs in line with the bench and your back straight.

2 Lower your body toward the ground, bending the elbows at 90 degrees, allowing the tricep muscles to engage. Push yourself back up to the start position, and repeat the sequence.

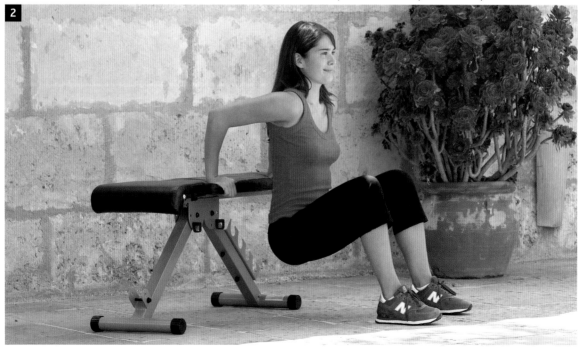

SUPERSET:
Preacher curl with stability ball 1 Set 12 Reps

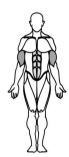

The muscles being worked are the biceps. Flex the muscles at the top of the movement. Concentrate on lengthening your biceps as you reach the start position

1 On your knees, lean over a stability ball grasping a dumbbell. Extend one arm over the ball, keeping your elbow soft.

2 Using your biceps, bend the elbow joint, curling the dumbbell toward you. Resist and control on the way down. Repeat the movement, then change arms.

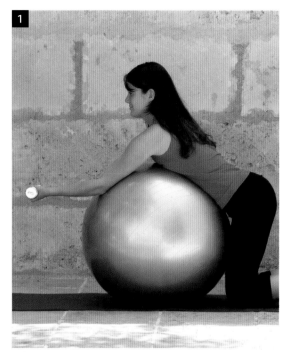

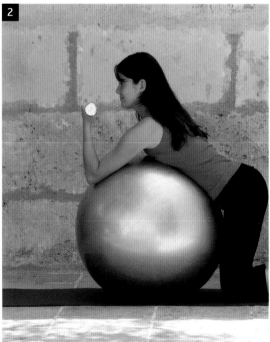

SUPERSET:
Barbell curl 1 Set 12 Reps

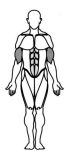

The muscles being worked are the biceps. Flex the biceps at the top of the movement and don't let those muscles rest.

1 From a standing position, left leg forward, right leg back, grasp a barbell, palms facing away from you.

2 With your elbows locked into your sides, curl the bar up toward your collarbone. Lower the weight under control keeping your elbows soft. Immediately return to the Preacher curl (page 96) and repeat the Superset.

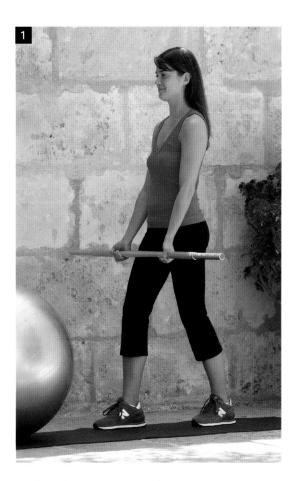

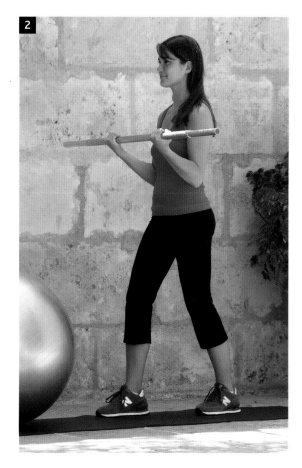

The clean 2 Sets 12 Reps

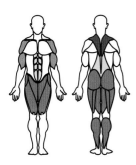

The muscles being worked are the gastrocnemius, quads, hamstrings, glutes, trapezius, deltoids, and biceps. Improve your technique before increasing the resistance. Concentrate on keeping your back straight.

1 From a standing position, grasp a set of dumbbells and draw your navel to your spine. Keep your stance at shoulder width, hips, knees, and toes all in line.

2 Bend at the hips and knees, and keeping your back straight, perform a dead-lift. Push upward through your glutes.

(cont. on page 100)

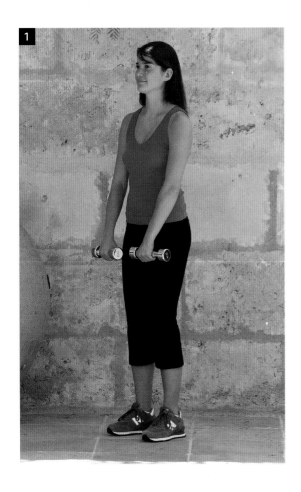

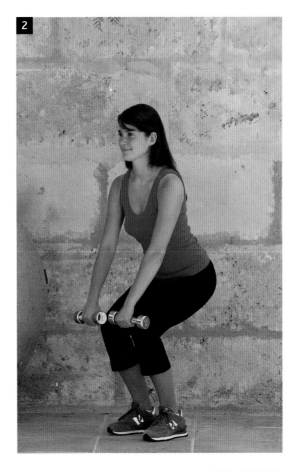

The clean continued 2 Sets 12 Reps

(cont. from page 99)

3 Rise up onto your toes and drive the elbows upward, performing an upright row.

4 In one smooth action, immediately rotate your shoulders, so that your palms are facing away from you, and your hands are on either side of your collarbone. Drop your heels to the floor and perform a squat. Return to the start position and repeat the sequence.

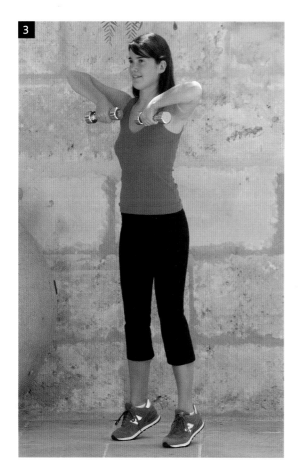

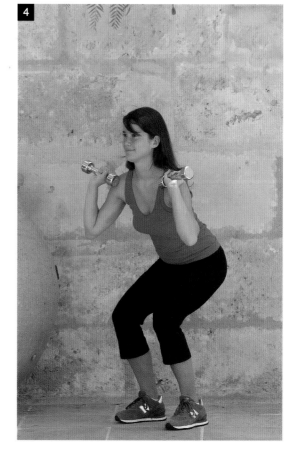

Ball twists 2 Sets 20 Reps

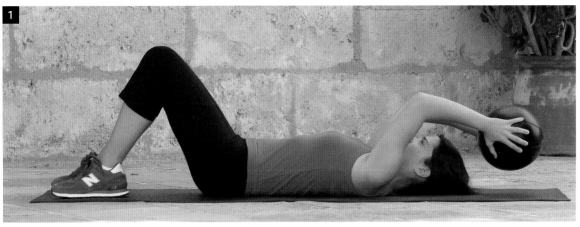

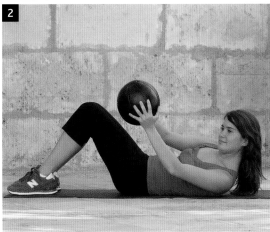

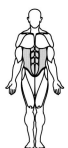

The muscles being worked are the obliques. Don't use momentum! Control the movement and grind out those reps!

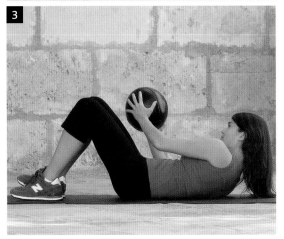

1 Lying on a mat with a medicine ball or soccer ball, start with the ball behind your head with your lower back pressed against the floor.

2 Lift with the abdomen, twisting to one side with the ball.

3 Lower slowly and repeat, twisting to alternate sides.

Stability ball crunches 2 Sets 20 Reps

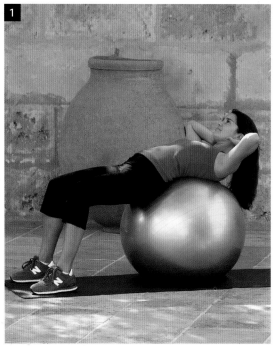

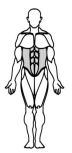

The muscle being worked is the rectus abdomen. Keep the movement smooth and precise. Try to close your eyes for added concentration and balance.

1 Sit on a stability ball and walk your feet forward. Lean back on the ball and activate your core muscles. Maintain a stable posture.

2 With both hands behind your head, curl your torso upward, shortening the distance between your sternum and navel. Return to the start position and repeat.

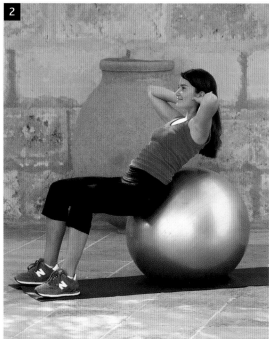

Reverse crunches with stability ball 2 Sets 20 Reps

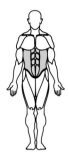

The muscles being worked are the rectus abdomen. Avoid arching your back. If this happens your legs have gone too far. Listen to your body and feel the muscles work.

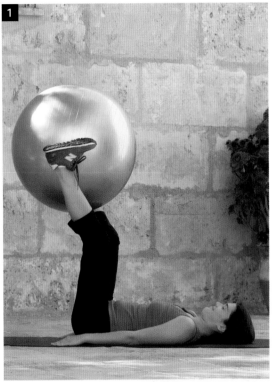

1 Lying on an exercise mat, place a stability ball between your feet. Place your hands flat on the floor on either side of you, with your legs up, feet facing the ceiling.

2 Moving from your hips, lower your legs away from you. Return to the start position. Slow movements are required, squeezing the abs throughout this exercise. Keep your lower back on the floor.

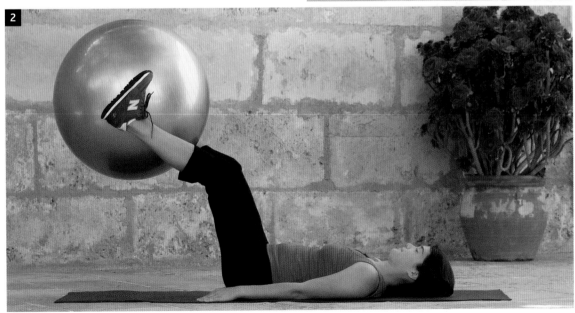

Advanced workout for men

Now 20 seconds rest is the max and go for it! Again, work with the same speed of the repetitions, 2 seconds up, 2 seconds down!

Knee dips   2 Sets 15 Reps

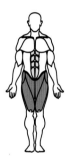

The muscles being worked are the quads. This exercise totally isolates the front of your thighs. Try not to stop when performing this exercise. Your goal is to get through all the reps in one go.

1 From a sprinter's position, heels against a wall, toes on the floor and in line with your knees and hips, slowly lower both knees until they align with your elbows. Activate your core muscles.

2 Push both legs up and back until extended. Under control, return to the start position. Try to keep the legs moving throughout this exercise. Stabilize your upper body.

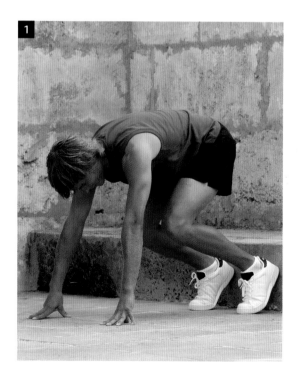

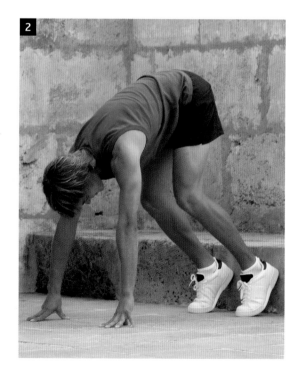

Four-point lunges 2 Sets 15 Reps

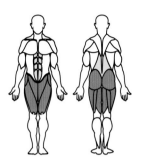

The muscles being worked are the glutes, quads, and hamstrings. Breaking the lunge down to four stages allows the individual to increase the weight.

1 From a standing position, grasp hold of a set of dumbbells, palms facing each other and draw in your navel to your spine.

2 Step forward with one leg and hold, making sure the rear heel comes off the floor. Bend at the hips, knees, and rear ankle, and go down into a lunge position and hold.

3 Press the leg back upward and hold. Now go back to the start position and change legs.

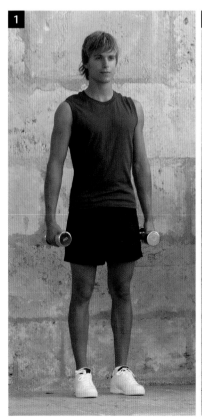

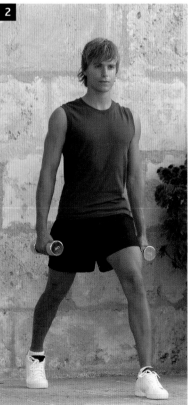

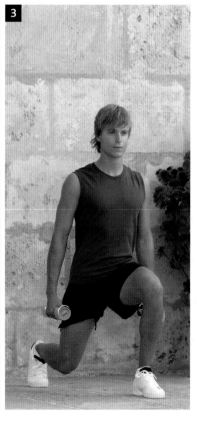

Ball squat 2 Sets 20 Reps

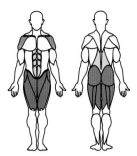

The muscles being worked are the quads, hamstrings, glutes, adductors, and deltoids. Keep your back straight throughout the movement. Try not to throw the ball too high and try to focus on the squat!

1 This is a total-body exercise with emphasis on your inner thigh adductor muscles. With your feet past shoulder width, make sure that your knees and toes are in line, and your toes are pointing toward 11 and 1 o'clock. Activate your core muscles. Holding a medicine ball or soccer ball, squat down under control, so that your thighs are parallel to the floor.

2 Throw the ball, allowing yourself enough time to stand up tall and then to squat down to the start position, catching the ball at the lowest point. Repeat the sequence again.

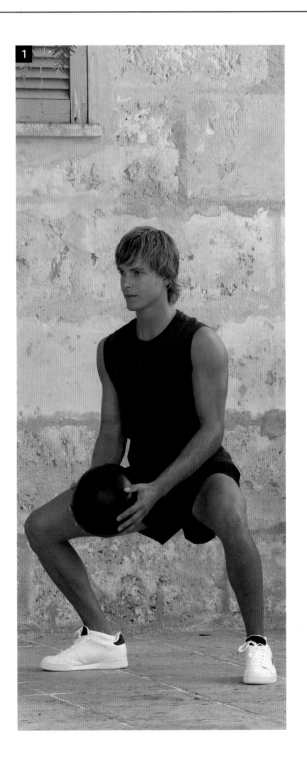

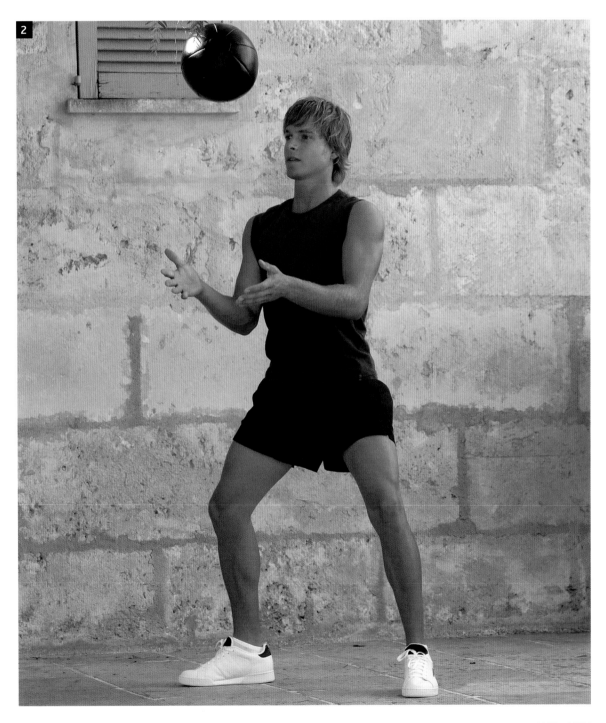

The clean 2 Sets 12 Reps

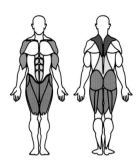

The muscles being worked are the gastrocnemius, quads, hamstrings, glutes, trapezius, deltoids, and biceps. Concentrate on your technique before increasing the resistance. Keep your back straight at all times.

1 From a standing position, grasp a set of dumbbells and draw your navel into your spine. Keep your stance at shoulder width, hips, knees, and toes all in line.

2 Bend at the hips and knees, and keeping the back straight, perform a dead-lift. Push upward through your glutes.

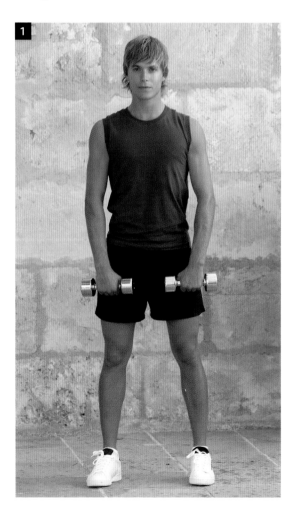

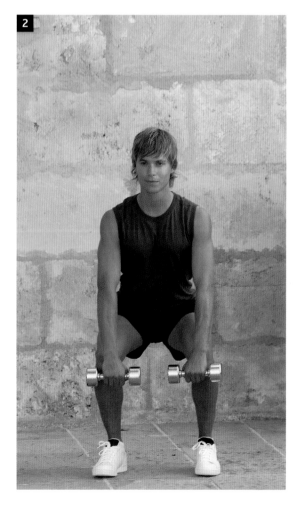

3 Rise up onto your toes and drive the elbows upward, performing an upright row.

4 In one smooth action, immediately rotate the shoulders so that the palms are facing away from you, and your hands are on either side of your collarbone. Drop your heels to the floor and perform a squat. Return to the start position and repeat the sequence.

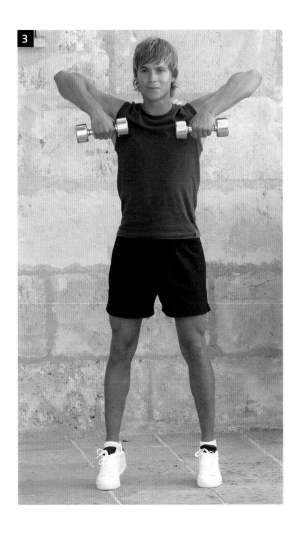

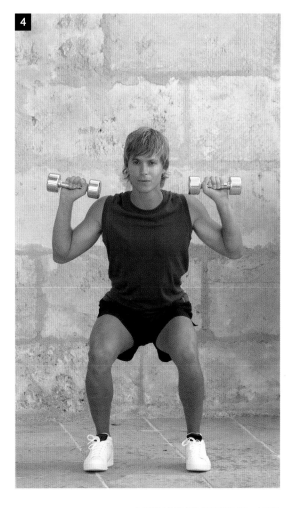

Reverse row to dead-lift with barbell   2 Sets 12 Reps

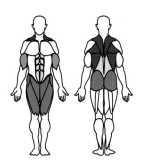

The muscles being worked are the latissimus dorsi, rhomboids, trapezius, biceps, glutes, and quads. I love this exercise! Keep the elbows angled and try not to round your back. Link mind and muscle, and isolate your back muscles.

1 With your feet shoulder-width apart, grasp a barbell with your palms facing away from you. Activate your core muscles.

2 Bend forward with your arms and back straight. Leading from the elbows, pull the bar in toward your lower chest area, squeezing the shoulder blades together.

3 Leading from the elbows, pull the bar in toward your lower chest area, squeezing the shoulder blades together. Now perform 3 repetitions. Push through the glutes and quads and stand tall. Repeat the sequence 4 times as one set.

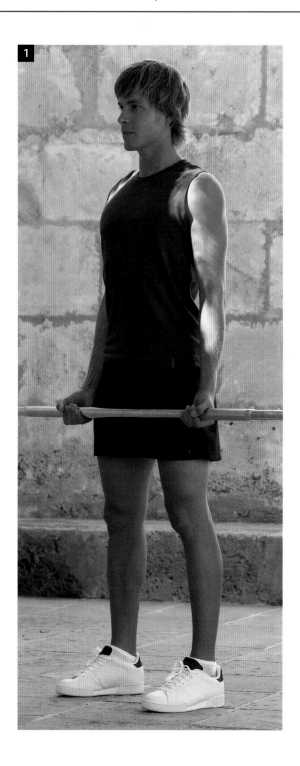

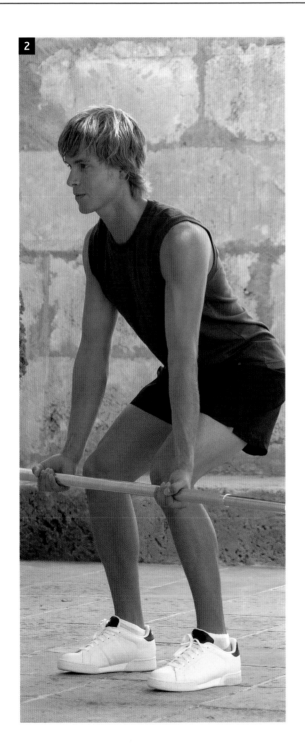

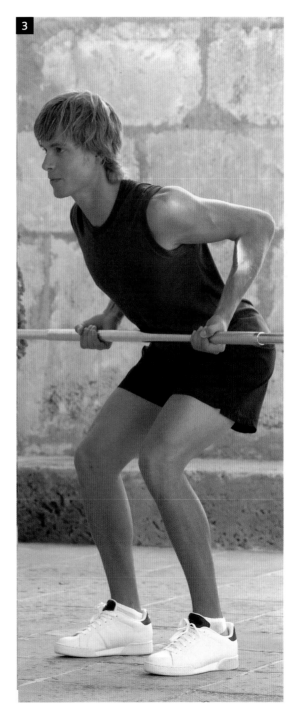

Cobra 2 Sets 12 Reps

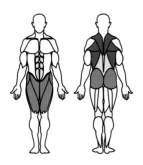

The muscles being worked are the glutes, rhomboids, trapezius, and lower lumbar. This exercise helps your posture and strengthens the muscles in your upper back between your shoulder blades and your neck.

1 Grasping a set of dumbbells, draw in your navel to your spine. Stand on one leg and lean forwards, keeping your back straight.

2 With your elbows soft, arch your arms backward so that the elbows are in line with your hips. Return to the start position.

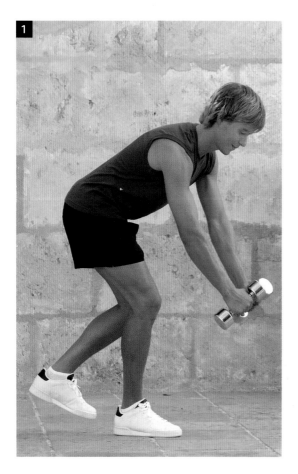

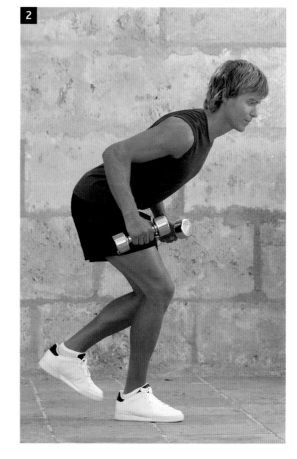

Rear shoulder flys with dumbbells 2 Sets 12 Reps

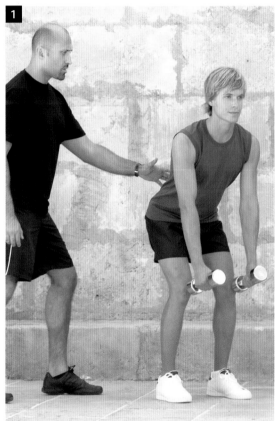

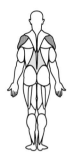

The muscles being worked are the rear deltoids. This is a fabulous exercise that works the upper back, with major emphasis on your rear shoulders. Avoid swinging your upper body. Stay with the 2 second up, 2 seconds down rule.

1 Activate your core muscles. Grasp the dumbbells, palms facing each other. From a narrow stance, lean forward.

2 Perform a flying action with the dumbbells, keeping the palms of your hands facing the ground. Make sure to keep the elbows soft, and raise the arms up to shoulder point. Lower the weight under control.

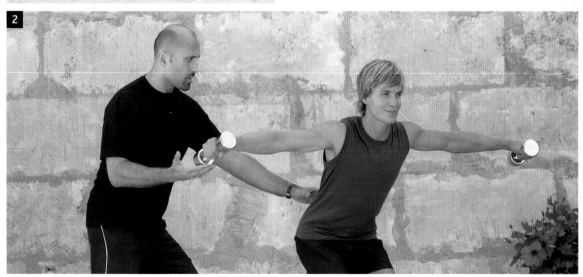

Two-arm chest press with dumbbells 2 Sets 12 Reps

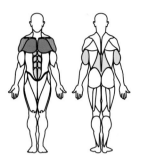

The muscles being worked are the pectorals, deltoids, and triceps. Press with your chest muscles. Try to avoid letting your arms do all the work.

1 Sit on an incline bench of 45 degrees and grasp the dumbbells with your palms facing away from you. Extend your arms with the elbows slightly flexed and in line with your upper chest. Activate your core muscles.

2 Lower the weight under control, so that the dumbbells reach the outside of the chest. Press upward and repeat the movement. Contract the chest muscles and rise to the start position.

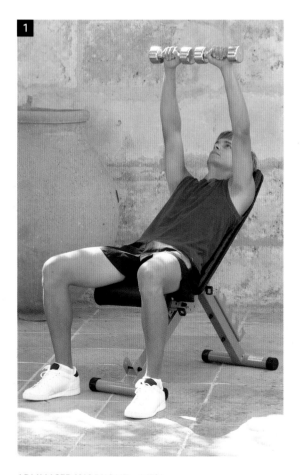

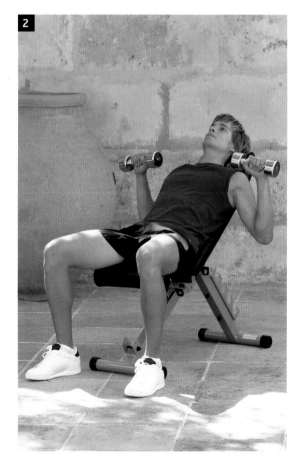

Flat-floor flys with dumbbells 2 Sets 12 Reps

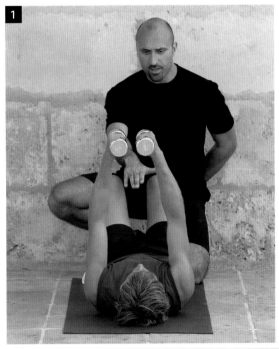

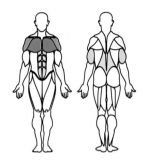

The muscles being worked are the pectorals and anterior deltoids. This is a great exercise for shape and definition of the chest. Feel the stretch through the pectorals.

1 Lying on an exercise mat with your knees bent, grasp the dumbbells, palms facing each other. Keep your elbows slightly flexed. Activate your core muscles.

2 Lower the weight under control as far as you can. Contract your chest. Raise the dumbbells to the start position.

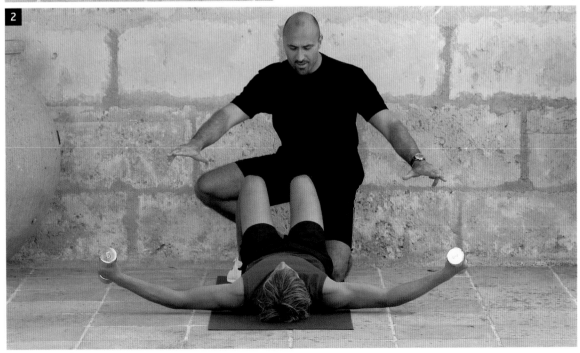

Unilateral standing raise with a dumbbell 2 Sets 12 Reps

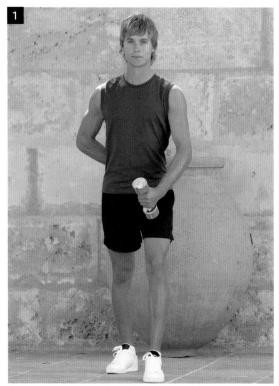

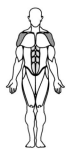

The muscles being worked are the medial deltoids. Try not to use too much weight with this exercise. The idea is to stimulate strong muscle contractions in the side of your shoulder, without the upper body moving. Feel the pump!

1 Grasp a dumbbell with one arm in front of you, one arm behind you, left leg forward, right leg back. Activate your core muscles.

2 Keeping the elbow soft, raise the dumbbell out to the side, until the upper arm aligns with the shoulder. Lower under control. Perform the repetitions then change legs and repeat with the other arm.

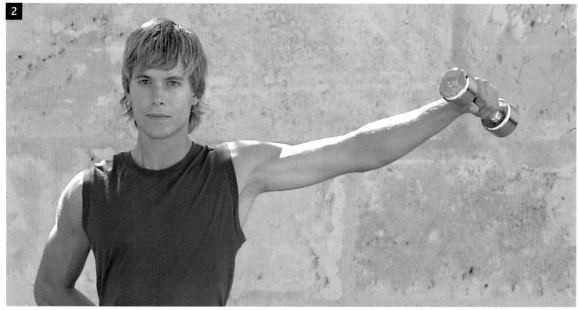

Two-arm upright row with dumbbells 2 Sets 12 Reps

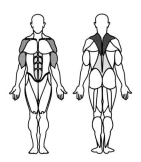

The muscles being worked are the trapezius, deltoids, and biceps. Drive those elbows up and feel your shoulders work. Don't stop now!

1 Using a set of dumbbells, arms at length and the palms facing you, put your left leg forward and right leg back. Activate your core muscles navel to spine.

2 Lead with the elbows and raise the dumbbells upward toward your chin, stopping at the collarbone. Bend the elbows and contract the deltoids. Lower the weight back to the start position.

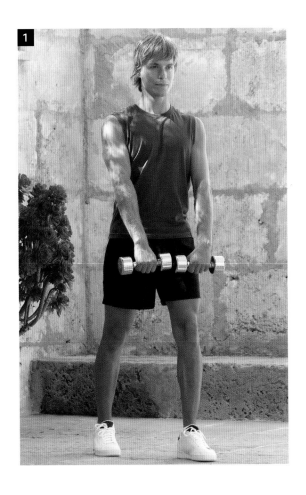

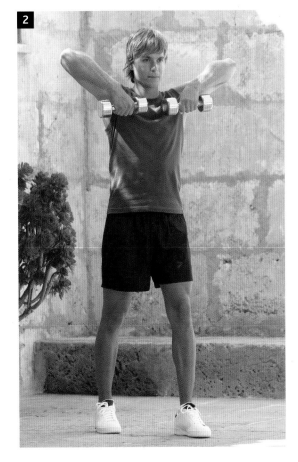

Incline triceps extension with barbell 2 Sets 12 Reps

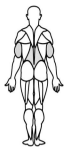

The muscles being worked are the triceps. This exercise develops them brilliantly. Go for it!

1 On a 45-degree incline bench, grasp a barbell. Position the hands so that they are two thumb-widths apart, with the palms facing away from you. Activate your core muscles.

2 With the arms at length, bend at the elbow joints, keeping the shoulders totally still, and allowing the bar to go just past your forehead. Press with the triceps back to the start position.

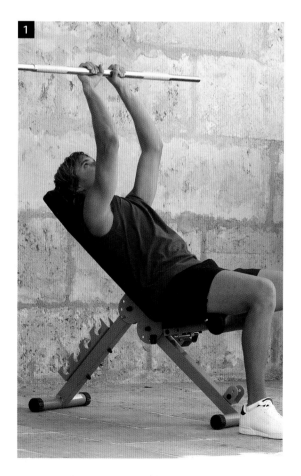

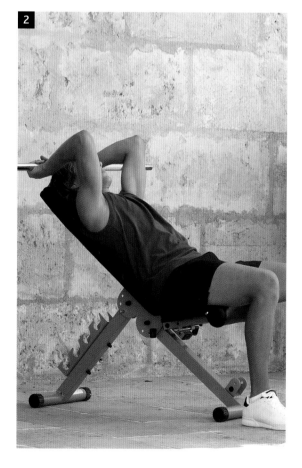

SUPERSET:
Incline biceps curl with dumbbells 2 Sets 12 Reps

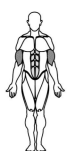

The muscles being worked are the biceps. Try to avoid letting your upper arm move and squeeze your biceps at the highest point. Feel the contraction.

1 On a 45-degree incline bench, grasp the dumbbells w.th your palms facing out. Lower your arms keeping your elbows soft.

2 Pull both elbows toward the side of your body and perform a bicep curl. As the curl reaches its peak, stop and return to the start position. Once 12 reps have been performed, move directly on to step 3.

(cont. on page 120)

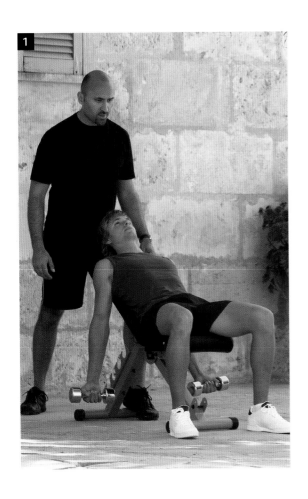

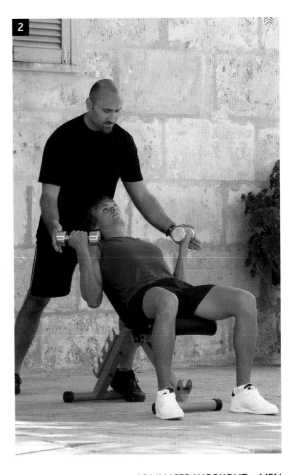

SUPERSET:
Two-arm standing biceps curl with barbell 2 Sets 12 Reps

(cont. from page 119)

3 From a standing position, left leg forward, right leg back, grasp a barbell so that your hands are in line with your shoulders, palms facing away from you.

4 With the elbows locked into your sides, curl the bar up toward your collarbone. Lower the weight under control, keeping your elbows soft. Once 12 reps have been performed, start the Superset again from step 1.

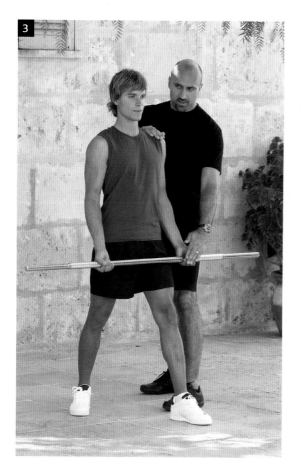

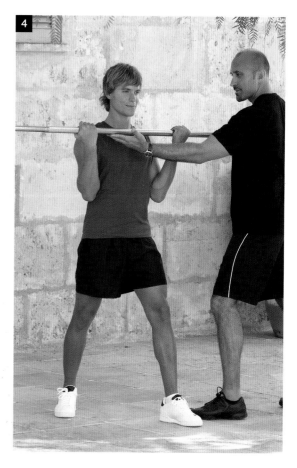

Advanced obliques 2 Sets 12 Reps

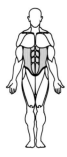

The muscles being worked are the internal and external obliques. Try to keep the straightened leg off the floor. This is such a great movement but very demanding. Keep your abs strong!

1 Lying on an exercise mat, straighten one leg 12in (30cm) off the ground. Bend the other leg at the knee, allowing the foot to touch the straightened knee.

2 With both hands behind the head, rotate the upper body, bringing the elbow across the body to knee point. Return, under control, to the start position and repeat the movement with the other arm and leg.

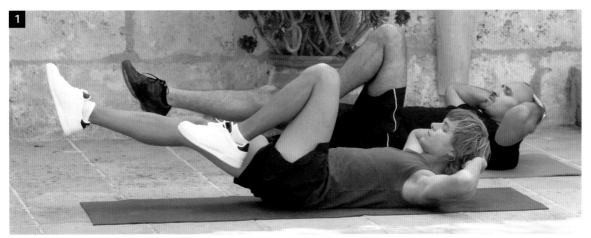

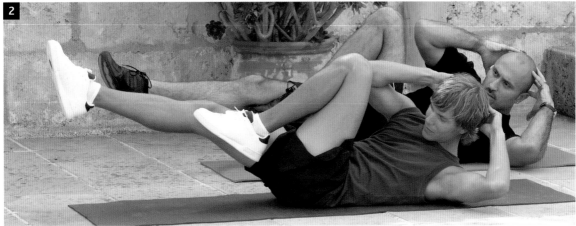

Crunch with stability and medicine ball 2 Sets 12 Reps

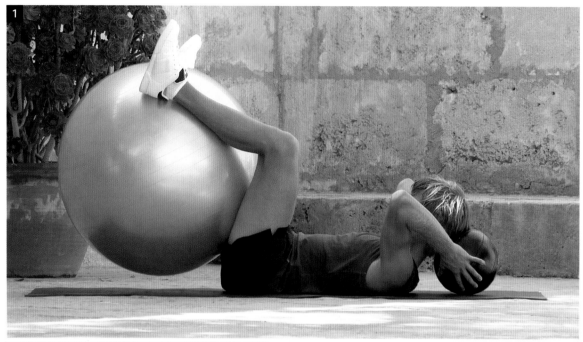

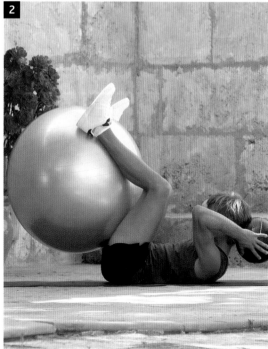

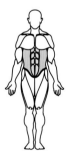

The muscle being worked is the rectus abdomen. Coordination is vital to achieve the full benefit from this exercise.

1 Lie down and hold a medicine ball behind your head. Grasp a stability ball in between your legs.

2 Raise your shoulder blades off the floor while lifting the stability ball toward you, using your abs. Return to the start position and repeat.

Plank on stability ball 2 Sets 30–45 second holds

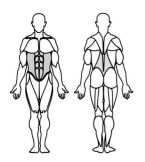

The muscles being worked are the entire core area.

1 With your forearms resting on a stability ball, hold your body up. Keep your elbows under your shoulder blades and forearms facing forward. Rest on your toes and keep your legs straight. Try to keep your body totally straight with this hold. Focus on pulling in your navel to your spine, and breathe normally.

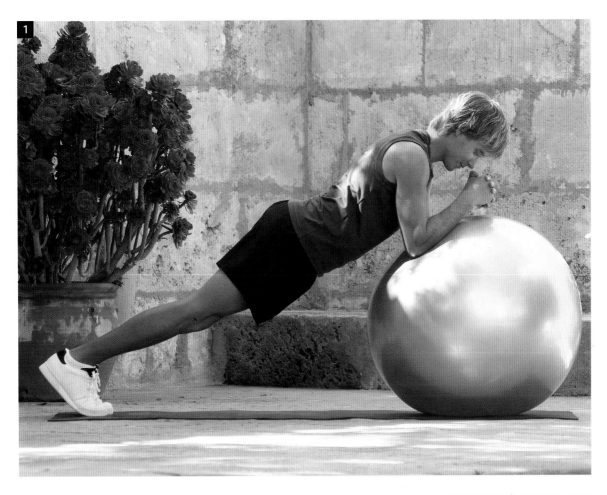

The cool down

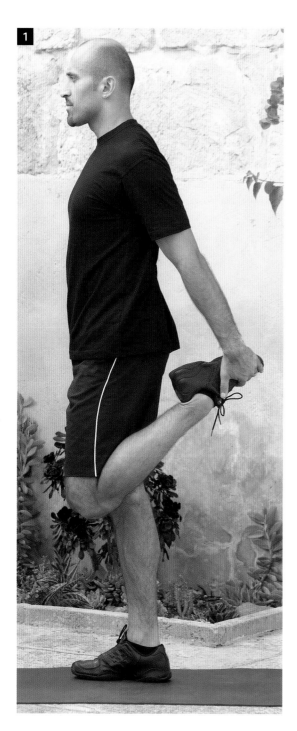

Cool down with a full-body stretch routine using static stretching. Each stretch should be held for at least 20 seconds, and as you become more flexible, start to increase the range of the stretch, and hold for longer. Stretching after exercise protects you from injury and improves the overall shape of your body by increasing the range of movement.

1 From a standing position, bend the left knee and grasp the foot. Gently pull the leg backward and feel the stretch in the front thigh. Hold for 20 seconds and change legs.

2 Take a wide stance, twice shoulder-width apart, with your toes pointing outward. Gently lean forward from the waist with your arms at

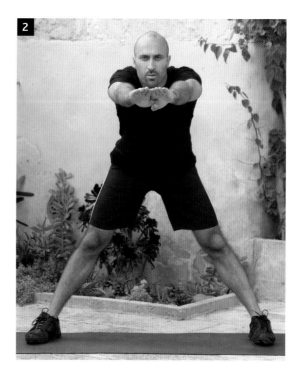

length. Relax and breathe normally. Feel the stretch in the rear thigh muscles and also to a lesser degree, the inner thigh muscles. Hold for 20 seconds.

3 Maintain the same stance, and place one hand on your upper thigh, and bend that leg. Keeping the other leg straight reach across with the other arm, feeling the stretch all the way down one side of your body.

4 From a standing position, place the palms of your hands on your lower back. Keeping the elbows angled, gently squeeze the shoulder blades together feeling the stretch in the chest. Remember to relax and breathe normally.

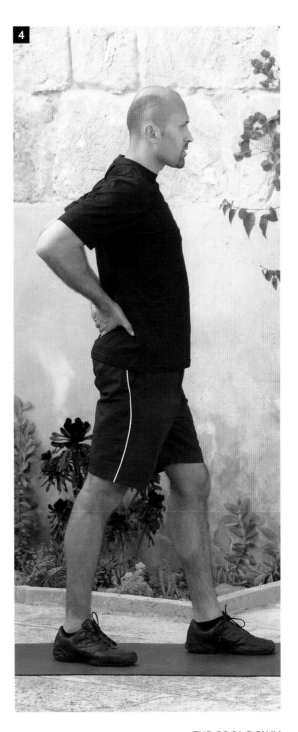

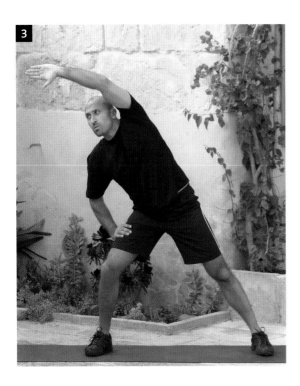

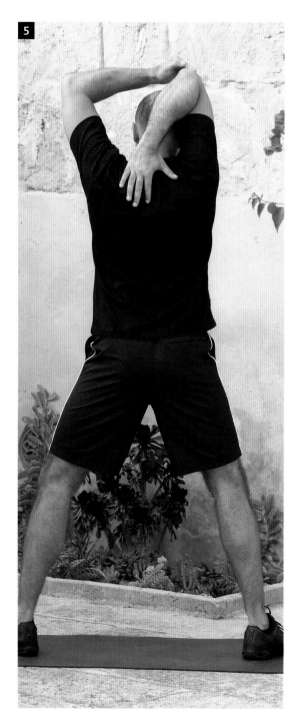

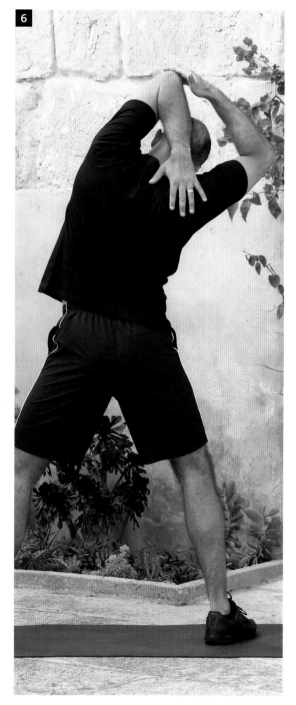

5 - 6. From a standing position, place one arm behind your head and bend it at the elbow. Make sure that the palm of your hand is in the middle of your upper back. Now place the other hand on the bent elbow, and press down. At the same time gently bend from the waist sideways allowing both the back and tricep to stretch. Hold for 20 seconds and change sides.

7 Rise up onto your toes and reach upward with your hands together. Lengthen the body. Breathe and relax. Well done!

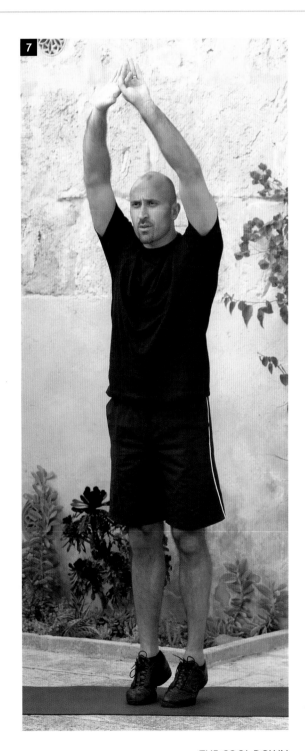

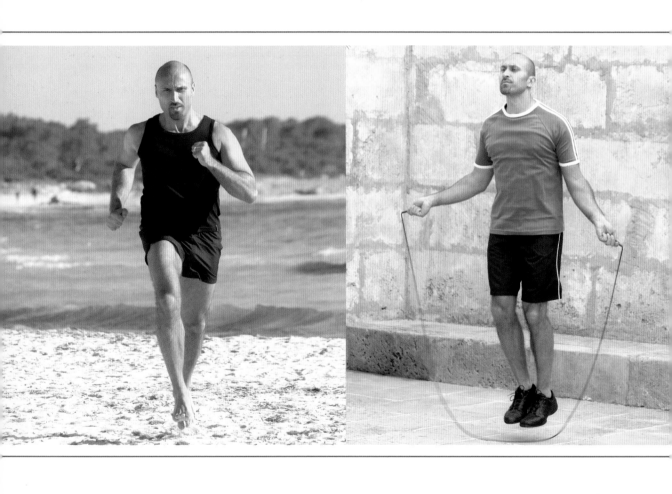

Cardio Work 3

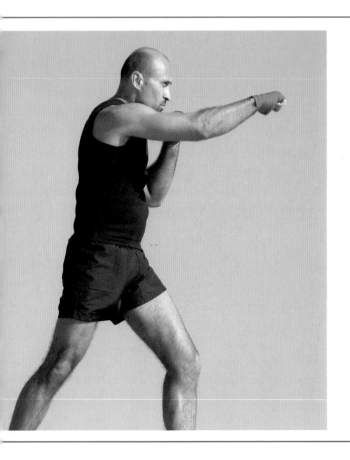

The overall feeling of fitness is something you just can't buy—it is the price of your time and effort. You must achieve a competent level in each segment of the fitness circle in order to successfully reach your goal of total fitness. Cardiovascular exercise incorporates stamina, speed, endurance, and coordination in equal measures. It also enhances fat burning. The most effective forms of cardiovascular exercise are running, power walking, shadow boxing, swimming, cycling, skipping, and for extra flexibility of mind, body, and spirit, yoga.

Your cardio options

Since the main workout is set at a high intensity level, aerobic workouts (or exercise with oxygen), should be done at a comfortable pace. However, the activity you choose will automatically increase in duration and intensity as you become stronger and fitter.

I always look forward to the long run I have with my brother on Sunday mornings. Every week it becomes easier and we're running faster, without causing our heartrates to go above 85 percent of our maximum levels. We couldn't believe it when initially we were hardly able to run 3 miles, and now we can easily smash 16 miles!

Each week, you'll notice this increase too, and it's so much fun if you do some form of exercise with a partner or friend. As you progress, it can lead to competitiveness between the two of you, which is a good thing!

To achieve increased levels in cardiovascular fitness, a minimum duration of 20 minutes is required 2–3 times a week. It is important to distinguish the difference between the once-a-week workout and your cardio activities. One high-intensity workout combined with 2 or 3 low-intensity activities is the right exercise balance in a week.

By combining your weekly workout with cardiovascular activity, you will increase your aerobic and anaerobic fitness. Because you're not overexercising, you are exempt from injury and fatigue. Your muscles will respond well to the right amount of exercise.

By doing other forms of activity you will help develop speed and agility, coordination and movement. Welcome to my training zone!

The graph shows that because of the increased fitness level needed to perform the Once-a-Week Workout, the cardio work becomes so much easier over time.

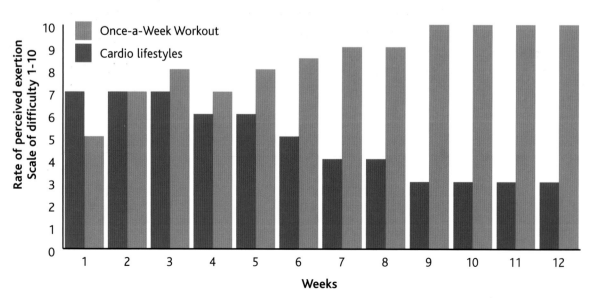

CASE STUDY 3: David Farr (34 yrs)

My name is David Farr, and I have been training with Mark for about 12 months now. I have found his program and training methods crucial for me to achieve my fitness goals. I had always been fairly sporty, and had trained both by myself and with other trainers over the past 10 years, but I had never made any real progress, and had become increasingly frustrated due to this. In fact, I had gone backward, I weighed well over 198lb (90kg), I am 6 ft 1, and was starting to fill out in all the wrong places.

I found the first few sessions with Mark challenging, particularly the short intervals between sets, and the outright ban on beer! After only a few sessions I began to see changes in my body as well as my fitness. I started to feel stronger, my recovery periods were much shorter, and I began to set personal goals on a regular basis. I was surprised at how quickly the changes occurred. In only a matter of weeks I had shed 11lb (5kg) and my body fat percentage had halved from 24 percent to 12 percent!

This progress has continued, and I am now in the best shape of my life at the age of 34. I certainly have achieved everything I initially set out to achieve, but have also surpassed my goals, and continue to set the bar higher every week.

I have learned a tremendous amount training with Mark. His regime of strength training, cardio, and diet, as well as his excellent motivational approach, has completely transformed my fitness, and has inspired me to set myself even higher goals for the future. I ran a marathon in 1999, and I wasn't in half the shape I am now. Iron Man, anyone?

MARK'S COMMENTS

David has worked so hard with me over the past year, and his results have been truly amazing! He now has the complete package: strength, stamina, speed, flexibility, and his nutrition has improved dramatically. His performance in the gym has blown me away! Chest pressing 290lb (130.5kg), compared to 70lb (31.5kg) initially! He performs leg extensions with 230lb (103.5kg), and lat-pull-downs with 310lb (140kg), and all during the same workout! His overall physique is just so different from the time he first walked into my studio. His relentless self-motivation helps him set personal bests on a weekly basis. Incredible!

"The mind is a powerful tool in developing the body through forms of exercise. It sets our goals for personal achievement and stimulates a strong working relationship with our muscles."

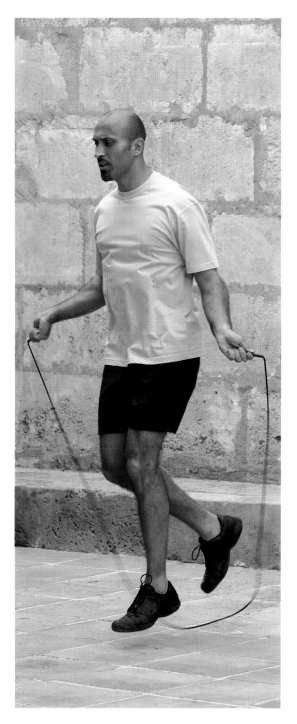

Skipping

Minimum duration 9 sets x 2 minutes

This is my favorite form of cardio activity. Skipping helps you free the mind and concentrate on balance, stamina, and coordination. Like anything else, with practice, you could be skipping for 20 minutes and beyond.

For best results, skip at an easy pace, keeping your arms out to the side. Make sure to keep the rope taught throughout the movement. The actual skip should be shallow and rhythmical. Aim for a 60-second skip initially; rest and try it again. As you become better at it, increase the time to 2-, 3-, 4-minute sets. You'll find that your body's ability to recuperate from exercise gets better and better.

A fitness circle week	
MON	Once-a-Week Workout
TUE	Rest
WED	20 min walk/run
THU	Yoga Class
FRI	Rest
SAT	20 min skipping
SUN	Rest

Running

Minimum duration 20 minutes

Sometimes, to really set you up for the day, or to put an end to a stressful day, a good, long, high-quality run is what you need. I look at it as my time of freedom! You're on your own!

Relax your shoulders, and allow your heart and lungs to work, so breathe constantly. Run at a steady pace without overexerting yourself, and go for distance and time. Try varying your weekly runs. If you run on a treadmill, add inclines and declines, slower pace training or quicker, longer strides for a faster run without causing breathlessness. Remember to stretch afterward.

Walking

Minimum duration 20 minutes

This is such an underestimated form of cardio activity. Without any change in diet, walking alone can help you loose 14lb (6.3kg) of fat over a year, plus, there's only $1\frac{1}{2}$ times the bodyweight going onto your joints, so this is good for everyone. Keep your strides long, with a heel-to-toe action, pull your navel into your spine, and keep your elbows close in to your sides and away you go. Let's rock!

Always stay well hydrated while exercising. It is a good idea to carry a water bottle with you, especially for long walks.

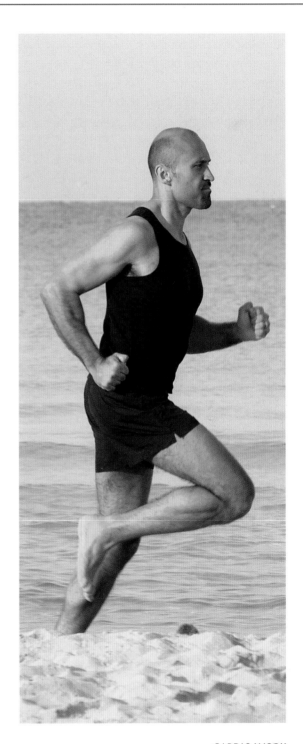

Shadow Boxing

This follows specific punches and body movements, using controlled and precise arm thrusts. The jab, cross, hook, and uppercut are involved with a small degree of kicking in this exciting new form of cardiovascular exercise.

Slowly build up to 7 sets of 3-minute rounds. Try not to use momentum or shadow box too hard, so that the workout becomes more aerobic. This form of cardio activity produces such an endorphin rush! It is one of the best cardio workouts I have ever had. You'll love it!

Yoga, Pilates, and Stretching

These are all gentle yet effective forms of exercise, which combine mind, body, and spirit, and are essential for keeping you supple, flexible, and strong. Flexibility enables us to perform tasks during the day much more easily. It is a great form of exercise to complete your fitness-circle lifestyle.

Other forms of activity can include swimming, cycling, team sports, low-impact aerobics, or even pushing your baby's stroller on a daily basis.

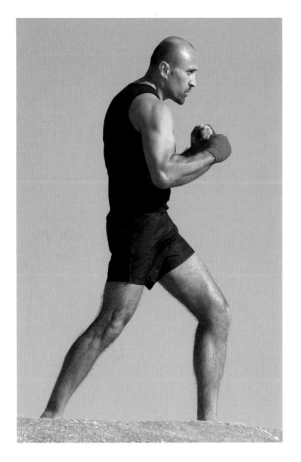

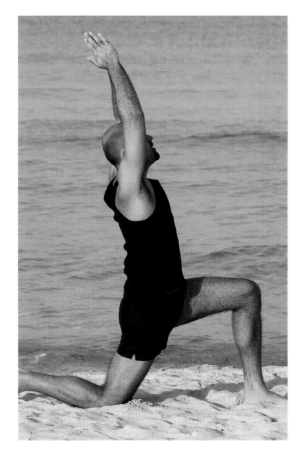

CASE STUDY 4: Jenny Borgerhoff Mulder (55 yrs)

My name is Jenny Borgerhoff Mulder. After spending the past ten years or so snowboarding, I decided to realize my "dream of dreams" and go heliboarding in the Himalayas with my husband. At the age of 55 I'm pretty fit, but not at all strong, and it was with a view to gaining strength that my Pilates teacher advised me to get in touch with Mark. I wanted to be as strong as possible, so as to face any conditions that may arise in the high mountains.

I worked with Mark just once a week, and did find our sessions hard work. But Mark is an encouraging, motivating, and friendly character, and it is his support that kept me going through each workout.

The results have been beyond anything I could have expected. Not only have I gained hugely in strength, which is what I set out to achieve, but as sort of an incredible free bonus, my entire body shape has also changed, which is quite amazing and unexpected at my age!

I am absolutely thrilled; this kind of training with Mark will play an important part in my future life.

MARK'S COMMENTS

Jenny's body changed very quickly: her commitment to exercise is a credit to her. She combines the once-a-week workout with walking and Pilates to complete her fitness-circle lifestyle. Her water intake is now exceptional, and she is careful with her food. The ability of her body to recuperate from high-intensity resistance training is now excellent, as is her health, body, and overall fitness. Jenny's body changed within weeks, so much so, that her friends and family noticed a huge difference very early on!

"Exercise is a release of mental and physical effort over a sustained period of time. One without the other is equal to zero."

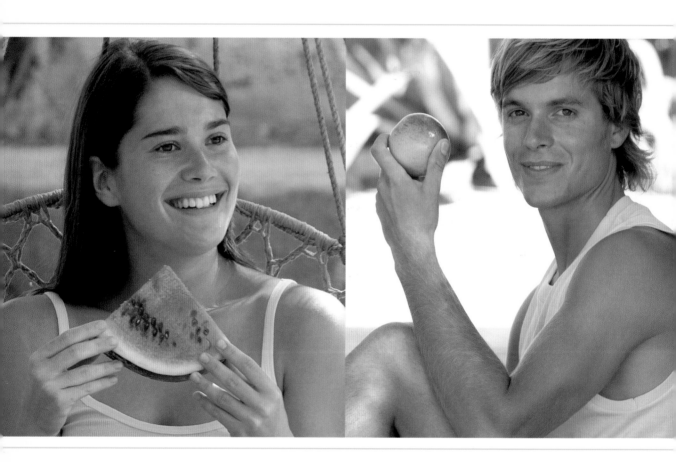

Eating Right 4

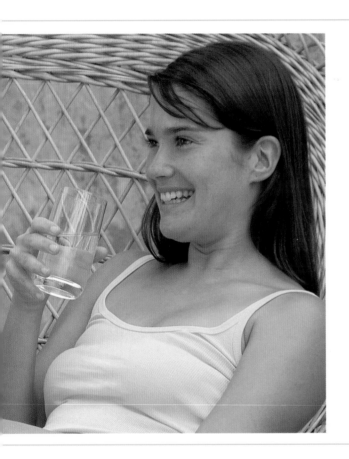

A good, healthy, and varied diet provides our bodies with optimum nutrition, which keeps us full of energy. Vitality equals happiness, happiness equals contentment, and contentment equals fulfillment. Breakfast is the most important meal of the day so don't skip it. Manage your portions and try to eat little and often. Eating right can play an important role in getting a good night's sleep, giving the mind and body a chance to rest and repair itself.

Healthy eating is healthy living!

Portion control is the best way to correctly measure food the body requires to function. Use the palm of your hand as a portion guide. One palm should equal a portion of protein, one palm a portion of carbohydrates, but two palms a portion of vegetables.

The body works best when you eat food in certain combinations. Our food for the day should consist of 50 percent carbohydrates, 25 percent protein, and 25 percent essential fats.

A certain amount of fat is essential in everyone's diet. Fats provide a concentrated source of energy. The body also needs to store some fat in order to prevent excessive loss of body heat. A certain amount of fat is essential in everyone's diet. Protein is needed for the growth and repair of our muscles. Food such as meat, fish, soybeans, and cottage cheese contain all the essential amino acids that are essential to our bodies. Carbohydrates provide our bodies with the main source of energy.

Mark Anthony's rules

- Never miss breakfast!
- Always buy fresh organic food.
- Avoid bread, butter, sour cream, mayonnaise, creamy salad dressing, desserts, and salt.
- Decrease alcohol levels to a minimum.
- Increase water intake to 2 quarts of uncarbonated water per day.
- Take water-soluble vitamins—B complex and vitamin C—to ensure adequate nutrition. These vitamins can be taken daily.
- If your body craves chocolate, have some, making sure it has a high cocoa content. After all, we have to enjoy living.

Diets too high in protein put an unhealthy strain on your kidneys and liver. Also the weight loss you experience is not all from fat. As your carbohydrate stores reduce, you begin to dehydrate and lose a lot of water weight. Your mouth becomes dry and your skin loses its suppleness. Because of the absence of carbohydrates, the body then metabolizes lean muscle tissue. Your energy is depleted and you

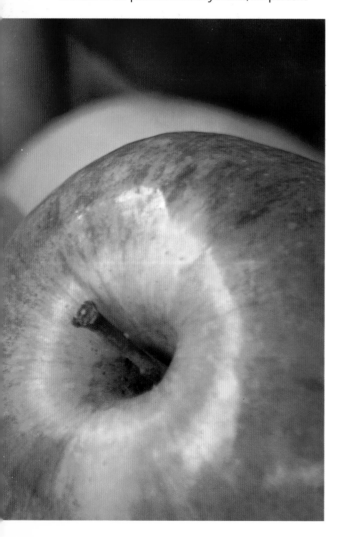

become drawn and tired. You are also prone to dizziness, nausea, and other symptoms.

Many individuals that I have trained were on a high-protein diet before seeing me. As soon as they started exercising, they would use up all the carbohydrate stored as glycogen in the muscles and feel totally exhausted within minutes. So a high-protein diet is not a healthy diet.

Water is by far the best diet pill. By supplying the body with 2 quarts of pure water a day it combines with proteins, carbohydrates, and fats and transports them through your body. Water also helps flush out impurities and toxins. It provides a healthy glow to your skin, and helps with the reduction of cellulite.

Suggested foods

- Avocado
- Cashew nuts
- Eggs
- Fish
- Soybeans
- Seeds
- Brown rice
- Potatoes
- Olives and olive oil
- Cottage cheese
- Peanuts and peanut butter
- Whole wheat bread
- Beef
- White meat
- Salad
- All fruits and vegetables
- All vegetables

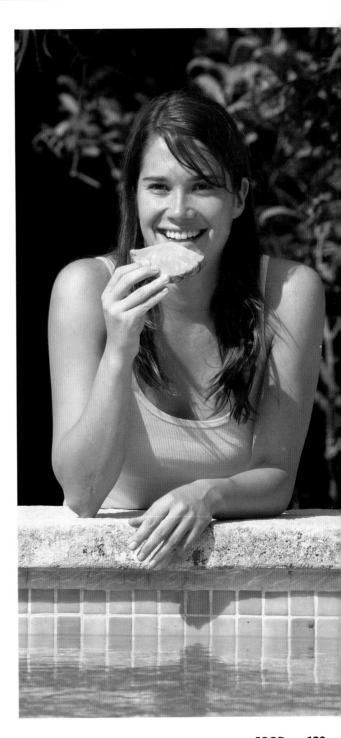

Moving on...

The Once-a-Week Workout provides 50 percent of completing the radical change in you. The other 50 percent comes from your commitment and dedication toward your overall fitness-circle lifestyle. Changing the human body isn't easy. There is always a degree of discomfort while working out, and also during the recovery stage. Hey, it's worth it!

By meeting me halfway, you will achieve so much more from the fitness-circle lifestyle. Increase your activity throughout the week, and make each repetition of each exercise count! You set your own standards each week, in terms of the intensity of the workout, and the resistance you use.

It's always a good idea to log your progress. Write down every single personal change on a weekly basis whether it's more repetitions on a bicep curl, more weight on a chest press, or more time on a treadmill.

Soon you'll want to feel a constructive ache in your body all the time. I always put it down to the fact that something is going on in terms of toning and change.

Remember to clear your mind of distractions, and anything else that stops you from concentrating. Stay focused on your goal.

Remember that the workout should be performed 12 times over a 12-week period, and at the end, if you've followed all of this, you will have successfully changed your body and your life. A winner never quits! And a quitter never wins!

My passion, energy, and belief in my concept enables me to set new standards when it comes to body change. Whereas at the beginning, on average, people changed after weeks 8/9, it is now, astonishingly, happening at week 3!

I'd like to wish you all the very best as you embark on this exciting fitness challenge. Although simple in theory, connecting the mind, muscle, and appetite, together with rest and recuperation, will provide you with more energy than you have ever had before. Yes; more energy for you to put into other priorities, such as family, social, and work life. Your confidence will improve, as will your zest for living!

The Once-a-Week Workout doesn't just end at 12 weeks, it becomes a continuous force of exercise throughout the rest of your life. Miss a week and you'll go crazy!

Follow the principles set out in this book, and take your body and fitness to new levels.

Become the person you want to be, and embrace change. Now work with me!

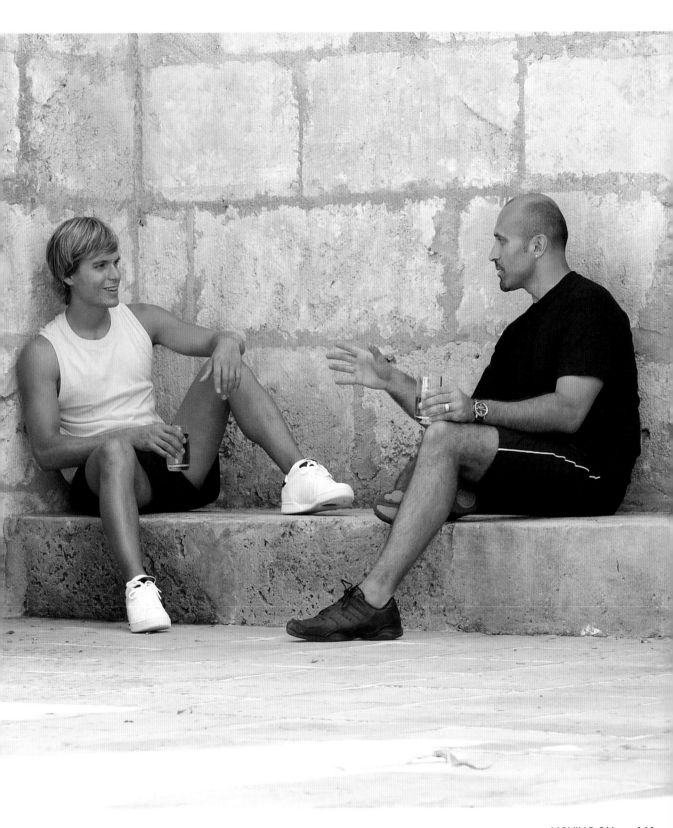

Training log

Photocopy this training log three times and use it for the beginner, intermediate, and advanced workout. List your excercises and write the weight you are using. Doing this will enable you to monitor your progress.

Resistance week by week

Once-a-Week Workout Name of exercise	Sets	Reps	Weeks 1	2	3	4	5	6	7	8	9	10	11	12
1.														
2.														
3.														
4.														
5.														
6.														
7.														
8.														
9.														
10.														
11.														
12.														
13.														
14.														
15.														
16.														

Optional Cardio Activities

Optional Cardio Activities Name of cardio exercise	Weeks 1	2	3	4	5	6	7	8	9	10	11	12
1.												
2.												
3.												
4.												

Index

Acknowledgments

With special thanks to Marcus Leaver for believing in me. To Dawn Forrester-Dorme for her relentless dedication to getting this project into the present book format, I truly thank you.

To the team at Chrysalis books, especially Victoria Alers-Hankey, for her commitment and enthusiasm for my book, and also for looking after me at a memorable stay in Majorca, thank you. Thanks to Gemma Wilson for the book's wonderful design, and to Guy "the doom" Hearn for the superb photos.

To all of our models, thank you for being so professional.

To Liz Puttick, my literary agent, my very sincere thanks.

To my father, thanks for giving me the best childhood any son could ever ask for. And, to my mother, whom I miss more than words can say, I wish she were still with us.

To my brothers Scott and Neil, thank you for the friendship we have together and the strong bond we have as family.

To all my family and friends, here's to the good times!

To all my clients that have put their time, money, and effort into my training ways, you are all champions!

And finally to my wife Gillian, I thank you for always being by my side since I met you 18 years ago. You are my one and only. During the past 10 years of my life, I have dedicated so much to personal training. This is for you honey!

To my superstar son Luke, and to my beautiful daughter Sophie, daddy loves you!